Thyroid Healthy

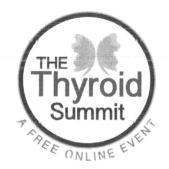

Join me as I host a worldwide event.
Listen to 30 amazing thyroid experts
with life-changing information!
www.TheThyroidSummit.com

Thyroid Healthy

Lose Weight, Look Beautiful and Live the Life You Imagine

Suzy Cohen, RPh

Cover Design: Batya Cano, GrafikaNefesh@gmail.com
Interior Design: Ronnie Moore, WESType@comcast.net
Photos: Melissa Shanley, MelissaShanleyPhotography.com

ISBN 978-0-9818173-6-1

Library of Congress Catalog Number: 2014938277

First Edition   10   9   8   7   6   5   4

Printed in the United States of America

A Word to the Wise

No comments in my book should be construed as medical advice. This book is not intended to treat, cure, or diagnose your condition. Please discuss and gain approval for any changes to your healthcare regimen, medications, or treatment protocol. Please be advised that suggested nutrients (and dosages where given) are intended as general guidelines and not right for everyone. Thyroid disease is a serious, complex illness that sometimes requires immediate medical attention. Follow your instincts and always comply with your practitioner's advice. You must accept total responsibility for your health regimen and every health decision you make, this book is strictly educational. Getting several opinions from licensed practitioners who have expertise with endocrine disorders is advised.

*To my good friends Richard and Jean Nickoloff
and
all the good people in the world who have served
our country and given from the heart.*

Contents

Foreword

David Brownstein, M.D.
Author of 12 best-selling books including
Overcoming Thyroid Disorders

Suzy Cohen's newest book, *Thyroid Healthy*, is a must-read for all. Thyroid illnesses are occurring at epidemic rates. Yet, many doctors in this modern age, do not know how to properly evaluate a patient for a thyroid condition. More often than not, it is up to the patient to take control of their health care decisions by finding a health care provider who will work with them to properly assess their thyroid function. This is where Suzy's book shines. It will empower you, the reader, to take control of your health and optimize the functioning of your thyroid gland.

The thyroid gland is responsible for producing thyroid hormone that regulates the metabolism of each and every cell in the body 24 hours a day, seven days a week. Little variations in thyroid hormone production have big effects on each cell and on how the individual feels. For the last 40 years, doctors have been trained to only evaluate a patient for a thyroid problem by ordering a thyroid stimulating hormone (TSH) laboratory test. In *Thyroid Healthy*, Suzy explains why the TSH test is not the best way to determine if there is a thyroid problem. She makes a clear explanation of the limitations of the TSH test and why it is important to look at other thyroid lab tests such as T4, T3 and thyroid antibodies. Furthermore, Suzy explains why the basal body temperature test should be part of a thyroid workup as it provides crucial information to fully evaluate a patient for a thyroid problem. Suzy explains very simply why the TSH test should not be used as the sole indicator of thyroid disease which is something few health care professionals want to tackle. *Thyroid Healthy* tells you exactly what you need to do in order to properly evaluate the thyroid gland.

Suzy, being a pharmacist and author of the best-selling book *Drug Muggers,* is well aware of the importance of supplying the thyroid with the proper nutrients to produce the optimal amount of thyroid hormone. Our food supply has become deficient in many crucial nutrients. Over the last 50 years, due to overuse of fertilizers and pesticides, we have depleted our soil of vital ingredients. During my career, I have tested thousands of patients for their nutrient status. I can assure you that the vast majority of people are suffering from nutrient deficiencies. Many of these imbalances can directly affect the functioning of the thyroid gland. Correcting these nutrient deficiencies can supply the thyroid gland with the vital ingredients it needs to optimally function. Suzy explains this concept in an easy-to-read style, which provides you with clear recommendations on how to properly use supplements to enhance thyroid function.

One of the thyroid gland's main functions is to regulate weight. We are suffering from an obesity epidemic. Nearly two-thirds of Americans are overweight and one-third are obese. The consequences of this are severe; we have tremendous numbers of people suffering from diabetes, hypertension, cancer, and other chronic illnesses. Why are we suffering from such an obesity epidemic? Suzy makes a cogent argument that we will only conquer the obesity epidemic when we properly diagnose and treat hypothyroidism. Following her recommendations will allow this to happen.

We are the wealthiest nation on the face of the earth. Americans spend more money on health care than any other country. However, we suffer from more chronic disease and obesity than any other people have ever experienced. I have no doubt that we are suffering from so many enduring illnesses because of nutritional imbalances, toxicities, and hormonal imbalances. A large part of why we are seeing so many sick people is because physicians are not listening to their patients and not properly evaluating and treating thyroid diseases. *Thyroid Healthy* was written to reverse this sad trend. This book will educate you and empower you to make better health care choices. I believe this book should be read by all medical students. Every time Suzy writes a book, I learn something. By reading *Thyroid Healthy,* you will learn how to optimize thyroid function.

—David Brownstein, MD
Author of 12 national bestsellers,
including *Overcoming Thyroid Disorders,
The Miracle of B12 and Iodine: Why You
Need It, Why You Can't Live Without It*

Introduction

We are all striving to live each moment to the fullest and get more comfortable in our own skin. I'm aware we are all dealing with life situations, and our health is the number 1 priority. If you don't have good health, nothing else matters a whole lot. I want to help you so much! I bet you've gone to the doctor and said, "I'm tired, depressed and heavier than I've been in years." The typical response from your doctor is, "Stop eating so much and exercise more." I'm very empathetic from having dealt with the crazy medical system myself so I hear you, I feel you and I wrote this book for you. Each tissue in your body has a different need for thyroid. This fact explains why you feel tired and cold all the time, while your hypothyroid friend can't lose 10 pounds and feels sad all the time. Your co-worker has hypothyroidism too, but she has 12 different symptoms!

I'm a mom, and a middle aged woman at the time of this writing. I've been through a lot in my life. Professionally speaking, I've been a pharmacist and natural health advocate for 25 years with a strong focus on natural medicine, versus prescription drugs which I was educated in. I'm also a Functional Medicine practitioner and have been for 15 years.

In order to lose weight, look beautiful and live the life you've imagined, you need to keep youthful levels of key hormones. At the top of the list is thyroid hormone. I know that because I have had to overcome low levels of thyroid hormone myself. As a pharmacist for 25 years, I can assure you medication treatment and testing for this condition has barely budged in decades and as a result, you are suffering needlessly.

Did you know that thyroid hormone affects every cell in your body? Most people think thyroid hormone affects the gland only, which is situated down low in the front of your neck. The truth is, thyroid deficiency causes symptoms that are so obvious that it's ridiculous to *not* get diagnosed properly if only from your clinical presentation. The most common symptoms affect metabolism and emotions. You gain weight, and your mood deteriorates. The next obvious sign is fatigue. You tire easily, and energy runs out faster than it used to for no apparent reason. You feel cold more often. You don't handle stress. You feel less attractive and cry easily. Things in your body stop responding the way they should and it's not because you're getting old. Thyroid disease can strike 20-something year olds, so this is not an old person's problem.

Your thyroid gland literally drives your health one way or the other. It can make you look like the woman on the left, or the right. You can see from the picture how important thyroid hormone is to your health. That's me, and the image on the left is about 10 years younger than the image on the right which was taken a few months ago. Improving thyroid function wiped years off my face and 15 pounds off my body. I was never very heavy, but that's still a lot of weight for a small 5'3" frame. I went from 125 to 110 and you can see the difference for yourself.

Today I have much more energy than I did back then, I sleep well and feel great for almost 50. I'm active in yoga and Zumba and always up for a hike around Colorado if you want to come visit me. Back in the old days, I couldn't exercise for very long, I had dark circles under my eyes and I wanted to lie down and catch a breather several times a day.

This went on for a few years, back when I lived in Florida. I recall telling a physician in 2007 that I was tired frequently, and before I could finish the sentence he offered me a prescription for Zoloft. I wasn't depressed, I was just tired and sleeping 9 hours didn't change it. If you know me, you know I'm really easy going and happy, and laugh easily, even to this day. To be fair, I worked part-time at the pharmacy, and was writing my first book, plus I was a full time care giver. I did feel pretty squeezed when it came to my energy reserves, but this kind of fatigue felt abnormal in a way that is hard to describe. I think you know what I mean, I just felt heavy, easily winded, short of breath, and I got dizzy doing certain dance moves in Zumba. My mind was always sharp like a tack, and during this time I found it hard to stay focused which was weird for me.

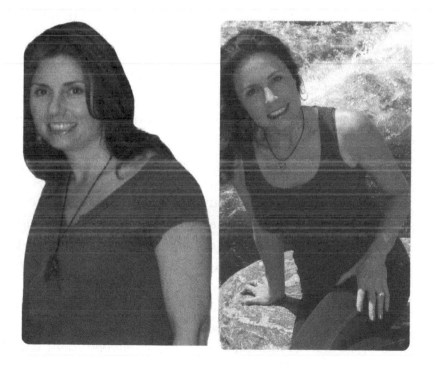

Anyway, when the doctor failed to recognize the true cause of my unrelenting fatigue and offered a mind-altering drug I knew I didn't need, I felt very alone and scared. *Is this going to be my life forever? Is this all my pharmacy has to offer?* At the same time, I was watching my sweet husband's health crumble despite interventions by dozens of doctors, he had Lyme but we didn't know it at the time, and the antibiotics he was given, actually poisoned his nervous system forever. You'll read more about those drugs later in this book. What a situation! It really made me think about my path in life, and how I would help myself and my husband. I vowed that if I could figure it out and get us well, I'd pay it forward. You are holding the result of my journey.

To keep the story short, I'll tell you that I eventually had my ferritin levels tested by another doctor. Ferritin is a marker of stored iron, and it was dreadfully low. It was 8, and it should have been between 70 and 90. My iron deficiency anemia was affecting my thyroid hormone, and causing fatigue. Ah ha! That was a major discovery because standard tests for iron and thyroid were "normal." All of this affected my adrenal hormones too, making some of them literally undetectable (meaning zero). Iron and thyroid go together like best buds and I'll tell you more about this connection in Chapter 14 Iron Deficiency and Chronic Fatigue.

There's more to my personal story. My husband Sam has imbalances with thyroid hormone from the antibiotics that poisoned his thyroid gland. We learned about it because he is always cold, especially his hands and feet. Granted we live in Colorado now, but he was freezing in 100 degree Florida! When we went out together, we'd get in the car, and then he'd sit inside the steamy hot car in our driveway for a few minutes before turning on the vehicle and air conditioner. He said the hot car felt good to him. (I was cringing the whole time because I hate the heat). I would sit for as long as I could tolerate it and as sweetly as I could muster, I'd blurt out "Turn on the freaking car!"

At a routine doctor's check up, we found out his body temperature was 94.8 at 3pm in the afternoon! We kept tracking it, and found that it hovered between 94.5 to 96.0. Normal body temperatures are about 98.6. *No wonder he wanted to sit in his vehicular sauna!* Now we live in Colorado, and we've purchased a real sauna so he can sit in that to his heart's content, instead of boiling me in our car.

You can imagine how every bodily system for Sam was compromised with a temperature that low. Your thyroid gland is one of the mechanisms in charge of your body temperature and sense of hot and cold. This information is not new, in fact, decades of research is available for you on Pubmed.com. You don't have to research yourself because I've done it for you. I'll share important life-changing tips from the literature I've pored through, and from well-designed clinical trials.

Some of the articles and citations I've used in this book are old. You may wonder why I chose to include old data. Instead, I want you to ponder this: *"If this data has been in the scientific journals so long, why have I not been told this?"* Sadly, it takes 20 to 30 years for mainstream medicine to incorporate new ideas. There are debates about how to test and treat a patient with thyroid disease. So many things in medicine become a very political or emotional debate with doctors who feel what they learned in school is absolutely correct. Sigh. They argue and you suffer.

The typical scenario goes down like this, your doctor orders a thyroid test, and when the results are within the normal reference range, you are told "Everything's normal, you're fine." But you know that you're not! You shouldn't have to look on 'Dr. Google' to find out you are hypothyroid when you are paying a physician to uncover this. One goal for my book is to give you mind-blowing information that you've never heard of before. I'll also offer simple solutions when I can, however I'm not going to mislead you into thinking that a "detox" cocktail will cure you, or a 3 day plan will solve 10 years of suffering. I'll never give you empty promises. Instead, I promise to give you hope and empower you with information about testing and treatments so you can uncover your true state of health. Remember, no two people are alike, so they can't be treated alike. We are all unique and our response to medicine and supplements is also unique.

Testing is a big deal because if I had been tested properly, I would have gotten better within months instead of dragging through my days for several years. The fact that you are probably hypothyroid and your test has not uncovered that just infuriates me. And it leaves you sick because you don't get the treatment you need. So the first point I want to make is that standard thyroid tests miss hypothyroidism up to 80% of the time! That's almost all the time isn't it? I'm validating you here and I believe you when you say your blood tests are normal, but you still feel like crap. Yep, been there, done that, got the T shirt!

The TSH (thyroid stimulating hormone) test is the one I'm referring to, and it's the first test ordered by physicians because that is the American 'standard of practice.' That's the lingo used to describe guidelines and principles that a doctor follows in order to treat patients. To offer other (better) tests for thyroid is not in keeping with the standard of practice, but I know excellent doctors who do it, while their peers stand in judgement. They're heroes in my book. Seeing a good doctor is the first step to getting well.

I'm honored that you have put your trust in me and I'm determined to hold your hand through this process. Nothing would make me happier than for you to live the life you imagine, one that is beautiful and happy, strong and healthy. You will have to find a doctor that believes you! I will teach you about labs so that you can get yourself tested properly. I'm going to teach you how to speak a thyroid 'language' so intelligently that you'll be taken seriously, and you'll be respected.

You have to become thyroid smart to become thyroid healthy! This means you will learn new concepts and at first they may seem complicated, but I'll keep repeating them throughout my book. I have videos at my website to help you understand everything that I've written here.

I have confidence in you. You deserve to enjoy a life that is energetic, healthy and happy. It's time to get thyroid healthy! For all the money you have spent on doctors, tests, supplements, medicine... my gosh, you should have felt better years ago! I promise to help you the best that I can. We're in this together, okay?!

Love,

Part I
Thyroid Basics

Chapter 1

One Gland with a Big Job

Your thyroid is a precious gland, you only have one. It's very fragile, shaped like a butterfly at the base of your neck and highly susceptible to chemicals in your pool, your toothpaste, your drinking water and even your new car. All sorts of chemicals can hurt your thyroid gland which is in charge of secreting thyroid hormone.

Thyroid hormone affects every cell in your body and you have trillions. Thyroid hormone regulates all of your activities, every second of the day. One of its main duties is to break down what you eat and create energy for you. Turn food into fuel. What if your thyroid isn't functioning well? You will obviously be tired. That is why a classic symptom of low thyroid is fatigue, especially morning fatigue. If the fatigue lasts all day, it's a sign of poor adrenal function along with low thyroid. When thyroid goes down adrenal hormones go up for awhile. When your adrenals start pumping out excessive cortisol from all your stress, you get inflamed and have pain.

When you have a thyroid gland disorder, it could mean that you have too little thyroid hormone (hypothyroidism), or too much (hyperthyroidism). An estimated 20 million Americans suffer from thyroid disease, yet 60% of people are completely unaware they have it. Women are dramatically more prone to thyroid disease. Some experts estimate that women are five to eight times more likely to develop it compared to men. Thyroid disease is always tied to adrenal fatigue and hormonal imbalances and you can see it in a woman's face quickly:

✓ Thin, dry hair
✓ Eyebrows may curve straight down on outer edges
✓ Hair missing on outer edge of eyebrows
✓ Lower eyelashes missing or sparse
✓ Cystic acne around mouth or chin due to hormonal imbalance
✓ Darkness on the inside corner of the eye due to adrenal fatigue
✓ Dry skin
✓ Puffiness around the Adam's apple

Because the symptoms of many thyroid disorders can be very subtle, they are often overlooked or mistaken for other health issues. I recommend that you have your thyroid hormones evaluated with a blood test annually. Many of you have hypothyroidism but it's not recognized. Have you heard any of these comments:

✓ You're just depressed.
✓ You're fat.
✓ You're going through the change.
✓ You're menopausal.
✓ It's all in your head.
✓ Stop reading Facebook, I know more.

When you don't have the support and help of an educated practitioner you continue to feel bad and relationships suffer. You could get depressed! You endure weight gain, or stubborn weight loss even though you eat very little. The way you feel physically and mentally taxes you. Worse, your course of action becomes blurred, costly, and frustrating. It's a derailment of life that I feel is repairable. Turning to forums on the Internet doesn't help because you read about what others did, but their path may not be right for you. The advice on the Internet can be misleading, incorrect or downright dangerous. Hypothyroidism causes every system in your body to slow down. The opposite is true for hyperthyroidism. Most people suffer from hypo, so that is the primary focus of my book. I have included a short chapter on hyper (Chapter 17, *Graves' Disease*) for completeness sake.

Are You Hypothyroid or Thyroid Sick?

This next section is HUGE news. I am making a distinction for you that should ultimately lead to your cure. Understanding what I'm about to tell you is important in speaking with your practitioners, and getting yourself tested, diagnosed properly and treated effectively. There is a difference between being hypothyroid and being "thyroid sick."

When your thyroid gland malfunctions and produces too little thyroid hormone, I'm going to call you "hypothyroid." This leads to all the symptoms listed in Table 1, Symptoms of Low Thyroid Hormone, page 7. Your gland is not functioning well, and therefore, not making enough thyroid hormone. The term "hypothyroid" is commonly used in medicine.

I have to make a distinction for you somehow. So, if your thyroid gland is healthy, and it is making plenty of thyroid hormone, but you still have symptoms of hypothyroidism, I'm going to call you "thyroid sick." You may read scientific literature and see the term "thyroid resistant" or "cellular hypothyroidism." That is what I'm referring to, but I'm calling it "thyroid sick" for ease of reading. In this case, your thyroid gland is healthy, and it is making thyroid hormone but that hormone is not getting into your trillions of cells. You want thyroid hormone inside those cells, not loitering in your bloodstream. Make sense?

I hope this makes sense. Why would I refer to it as hypothyroid when your gland is pumping out plenty? I won't, I'll call you "thyroid sick" to make the distinction that you can have a perfectly healthy thyroid gland, and still have all the clinical manifestations of hypothyroidism because your hormone is not getting inside your cells. Your cells organize themselves to form your tissues which make up your organs. So what I'm saying is that being thyroid sick means you're cells are starving for thyroid hormone, therefore your organs are. And that can very well happen even though your gland is healthy and making plenty. You are not hypothyroid, technically speaking, but in my book you ARE thyroid sick. Most of you reading my book fall into the latter group.

Thyroid Hormone Production

Thyroid hormone production happens within seconds, and all the magic happening takes place just inches apart, yet it controls all 5 or 6 feet of you! Your hypothalamus (in your brain) produces a compound called TRH (thyrotropin releasing hormone) also known as protirelin, which signals your pituitary gland at the base of your brain to release another compound called TSH (thyroid stimulating hormone). So the TRH makes you churn out TSH. The TSH stimulates your thyroid gland to release T4 (thyroxine). The T4 hormone is not active in terms of making your thyroid hormone. T4 is not really a do-nothing hormone, it's "active" in the sense that it helps your body make a form of riboflavin called "flavin adenine dinucleotide" or FAD that helps you methylate. This FAD form of riboflavin reduces blood pressure better than a prescription drug according to one study. You need adequate amounts of thyroxine to create this FAD and use it for methylation. When you methylate you 'take out the garbage' from your body.

So we can't use thyroxine (T4) to wake up, but we can certainly use some of it to help us with methylation which takes out poisons from our body. Hypothyroidism automatically means less thyroxine, and less detoxification. In terms of feeling great, we need to wait for T4 to turn into T3 and it's that hormone that wakes us up. Therein lies one big problem with your health.

You hope it converts and activates itself to the form called T3 hormone, but if it goes another direction and forms Reverse T3 (rT3) it's a problem! This rT3 blocks the real T3 thyroid hormone from working, and then you're going to look like the poster child for hypothyroidism. Standard labs will all appear normal, because your thyroid gland is healthy, but you'll be face-planted on the couch, gaining weight without eating. You'll wash your hair and find wads of it in the drain. You're cold. Your cells are starving for thyroid hormone. You are thyroid sick!

Table 1. Symptoms of Low Thyroid Hormone

Apathy
Anxiety
Cold hands and feet
Concentration difficulties
Constipation
Depression
Disturbed sleep patterns and/or insomnia
Dry skin and hair
Fatigue or weakness
Hair loss or thinning on head
Hair missing on outer edge of eyebrows
Lower eyelashes missing or sparse
Heavy menstrual flow
Infertility
Joint pain
Low body temperature
Memory problems
Migraine
Muscle pain
Pale skin
Reduced ability to sweat
Shortness of breath with little exertion
Water retention
Weight gain or difficulty losing weight

Why Are We Being Misdiagnosed?

There's an epidemic of people who are thyroid sick (but not hypothyroid because their gland works) and they are being misdiagnosed. Are you one of these people? Physicians assume you are "stressed out" or depressed. The reason for the inability to have thyroid disease diagnosed correctly is due to the widespread use of a standard thyroid blood test called the "TSH" which stands for thyroid stimulating hormone. TSH hormone is a brain hormone that tells your thyroid gland to get off it's butt and start working. Think of it this way, your gland goofs off unless it gets yelled at to work (by TSH which comes out of your pituitary in your brain). The pituitary gland is a tiny organ, about the size of a pea!

A "normal" TSH value doesn't say much. But an abnormal value says a lot. Problem is, it takes a long time for the TSH to become abnormal, and you will be miserable by the time your TSH falls out of the normal reference range on a lab test. I'm telling you big news, do not rely solely on the TSH test. If you're uncomfortable and have all the signs and symptoms of low thyroid, despite a normal test, that's really common.

If your TSH falls within "normal" limits, you are told you're not hypothyroid. That part is true, but you could be thyroid sick ... and you often are! You could be dreadfully low in thyroid hormone inside a trillion cells. As I've just taught you, a person who is thyroid sick has every single symptom as a person who is hypothyroid! This is HUGE news. I want you to see that you can be clinically hypothyroid inside every cell of your body, but your TSH test could be normal. Only when you are severely thyroid sick, does the TSH move into the abnormal range on a lab test. By then you are super messed up, your relationship may be ruined, you may be on a medication merry-go-round and wondering how the heck did I wind up like this. Now you know, it's because the standard test for thyroid doesn't capture the happenings inside the cell, it reflects brain levels, not tissues and organs that are starving.

Why, Why, Why?!

The normal reference range for the TSH tests were established a long time ago. The range is based upon samples from very thyroid sick individuals. So from now on, I want you to assume the normal range to be much lower than what you see on your lab paperwork. The numbers keep changing, and differ from doctor to doctor, lab to lab. Some experts say a TSH above 4.5 or 5 is bad and requires treatment, but I personally think a TSH above 1.0 will make you feel bad. Most experts feel that a TSH somewhere between 1 and 2 is the goal, but I would never, ever depend on the TSH as my sole test.

If you're thyroid sick based upon your symptoms, and your physician stubbornly adheres to your TSH lab test telling you that you're okay because you are in the "normal" reference range, (and like I said, these are far from "normal"), this indicates he/she is not fully educated on thyroid disease or treatment. There are better ways to diagnose thyroid disease using the lab tests I recommend in Chapter 5, *The Best Lab Tests*. For me, it's really about how you feel. If you have a TSH of 3 and you feel great, let it be. If you have a TSH of 1.5 and you feel horrible, get treatment. We are all unique. The number one thing is to be gentle on yourself. Stop berating yourself for how you feel, and look, and all that you didn't do today because you were tired. Be gentle and loving to yourself.

To help you, I've crafted a "Script" for your gentle healing process. It's a plan to help you live thyroid healthy. As you continue reading the book, you will see me refer to this "Script" at times. In Chapter 24, *Live Thyroid Healthy,* I elaborate on each part of this S-C-R-I-P-T:

See a good doctor. Stop banging your head. Find someone who can test you correctly and prescribe or recommend medicine or supplements that work.

Convert T4 to T3. Improving conversion gives you more active thyroid hormone. T4 hormone (whether you make it naturally or take it as levothyroxine) does not provide active hormone, you have to convert that molecule to T3 to feel well. Most people can't effectively do that because of nutritional deficiencies or high cortisol, or low vitamin D or something else. Regardless of why, you will be hypothyroid despite normal blood tests unless you convert T4 to T3. It's huge.

Restore mugged nutrients. You're being nutritionally robbed by medicine, food and beverages. When you drink coffee, you lose magnesium and iron. When you take cholesterol pills, you lose vitamin D and CoQ10, when you take steroids, antacids or hormones, you lose zinc, selenium and other nutrients. This 'drug mugging' of your nutrient stash cripples your ability to make thyroid hormone.

Interpret tests correctly. If you accept the "normal" values on your test, you'll remain sick. The reference ranges today are not designed to advance your health, and if you abide by some of them, you will be hypothyroid forever. I want to enlighten you to the fact that your black and white lab results might say "normal" but those ranges are not trustworthy, they were based on sick people, not healthy ones. Why would you want to match up with that?!

Protect your thyroid gland from poison- When I say "poison" I mean certain food antigens that inflame your thyroid gland. Soy, gluten, dairy, refined sugar and artificial ingredients create a little metabolic fire in your body. The partially digested food particles make your internal chemistry go nuts causing your cells to spill excessive amounts of naturally-occurring compounds, but still, excessive amounts cause tremendous pain and inflammation as well as neurological, emotional and mental problems. Other "poisons" I want you to protect yourself from include chloride, fluoride and bromide found in every day products and foods.

Transport thyroid hormone. If you can't get thyroid hormone INTO your cell, you'll by hypothyroid. Once you have your thyroid gland protected and your T4 is converted into the form called T3, you need to be able to move it into the cell, specifically inside the mitochondria "motors" which give you energy. Transport of thyroid hormone is an active dynamic process. Thyroid goes in and out of the cell, all day long and the process is taking place thousands of times while you read this sentence. The transportation system cannot be clogged up like it is on 5th Avenue in New York City! Ever been there? It's a sea of yellow taxi cabs for miles, all honking. Why do they honk, there is no where to go, the cabs just sit there. You want the traffic of your thyroid hormone to flow, you don't want it stuck. Transport mechanisms have to be in order and there are nutrients and lifestyle factors that improve this.

Chapter 2

Thyroid Hormones Control the Show

There are many players involved when it comes to producing and utilizing thyroid hormone. The pituitary gland and your thyroid gland work together but it's the thyroid gland that makes and releases your hormones. When things go off without a hitch, the thyroid hormone gets transported into your cell and activated from thyroxine (T4) to a form called triiodothyronine (T3) that makes you feel great. In fact, just look at all the wonderful things thyroid hormone does:

✓ Regulates your heartbeat
✓ Warms you up
✓ Speeds metabolism so you lose weight
✓ Improves muscle strength
✓ Replenish dying cells with healthy ones
✓ Grows your hair and nails
✓ Gives you regularity
✓ Improves your ability to conceive
✓ Reduces sensations of pain
✓ Makes you feel happy and content

You can see from this list that thyroid hormones really do control the show! One issue with production, transportation into the cell, or activation and "we have a problem in Houston!" In order to make thyroid hormone, your gland needs tyrosine which is an amino acid, and it needs iodine atoms. The tyrosine and iodine hook up together and form thyroid hormone. That's what the "T" stands for, tyrosine. And the numbers like 3 or 4, mean the number of iodine atoms attached. So T4 hormone means a tyrosine attached to 4 iodines. And T3 hormone means a tyrosine attached to 3 iodines.

Conversion of Thyroid Hormone

In order for T4 (inactive) to become T3 (active), it has to be converted in a biochemical reaction. The conversion takes place primarily in your liver, but also in your kidneys, brain, gut and other organs. Specific deiodinase enzymes are necessary for conversion, which you will learn about later in this chapter. These enzymes chop off an iodine from T4, and thus produce T3, and then the party starts. Remember, T3 is what you need to wake up, look good, be happy and feel alive.

Figure 1

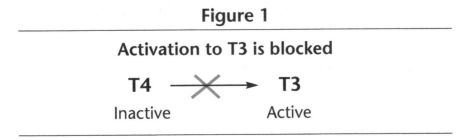

Activation to T3 is blocked

T4 — T3
Inactive   Active

So when doctors measure T4 levels in your body, it's not saying what is inside the cells and remember it's what's inside your cells that matter most. T4 doesn't even work, it is a pro-hormone. It has to become activated by dropping one of those four iodine atoms in a biochemical process called "deiodination." Nutrients such as B vitamins and minerals are needed for you to have adequate active thyroid hormone. You need selenium for the enzyme to work, and activate your thyroid. More specifically, you need selenium to make the enzyme that converts inactive T4 to active T3. Yeah, it's a big deal! Things are more complex than I'm saying here, but that's because I don't want to bog us down. Thyroid hormones can be metabolized in peripheral tissue by deiodination, deamination, conjugation, and decarboxylation enzyme reactions, but again, I'm not going to bog us down with these details because I know you really just want solutions, not science.

Synthroid is Pure T4

Your thyroid gland produces the natural hormone called thyroxine or T4. T4 is also sold as the popular prescription drug Synthroid or it's generic Levothyroxine. The medications are bio-identical to your own thyroid hormone. Whenever you see "T4" in the literature, or in my book, you can imagine it's acting just like your medication.

To become activated, T4 (thyroxine) must morph into T3 (tri-iodothyronine) and this, in turn, must find its way into the cells to do its work. Many things can go wrong with this process, often it is a deficiency in B vitamins, vitamin D or minerals which causes sluggish conversion of T4 to T3. The minerals are truly crucial, so eating mineral-rich foods can help you. Some people have a genetic polymorphism (mutation in genetic code) that causes impaired thyroid function. Whatever the reason, not having enough T4 to T3 conversion means you are clinically hypothyroid or what I call "thyroid sick." This is often overlooked because doctors are busy measuring TSH (thyroid stimulating hormone), a pituitary hormone that has nothing to do with what's happening inside your cells! All of the following improve the conversion of T4 to T3:

✓ B complex
✓ Vitamin D
✓ Magnesium
✓ Folate
✓ Selenium
✓ Zinc
✓ Ashwagandha
✓ Mullein herb

Let's Meet the Family!

TSH   Secreted by your pituitary gland that instigates
       thyroid production
T1   A hormone precursor or by-product, function not
       yet known*
T2   A hormone precursor or by-product, fairly weak*
T3   Triiodothyronine, the active thyroid hormone that
       you want
T4   Thyroxine, secreted by your thyroid gland and
       stored until needed (inactive)
rT3   Reverse T3, the mirror image of T3, non-functional
TPO   An enzyme often high in autoimmune thyroid
       conditions
Tg   Thyroglobulin, antibodies to this attack your
       thyroid (Hashimoto's)

---

*T1 and T2 are often dismissed because we don't know their complete function. These are both found in glandulars such as the prescription Armour Thyroid and I am convinced that one day, as research progresses, we will find out there was more to T1 and T2 than we know now. The big players in your body are T4 and T3.

More than 90% of the thyroid hormone produced is actually T4 (inactive storage form) and 7% is T3 (the active form). The inactive T4 has to be processed in your liver into the active form

T3. Under normal circumstances about 40% of available T4 is converted into the active T3 hormone. Some of it, about 20% gets activated in your gastrointestinal tract, compliments of a healthy microflora ... yes the beneficial gut bugs (probiotics). Lack of beneficial bacteria in the bowel can result in you losing 20% of your T3 thyroid hormone.

TSH or Thyroid Stimulating Hormone. It goes by "Thyrotropin" sometimes. It's produced in your pituitary gland in your brain. It's sometimes referred to as a "brain" hormone but to be technically correct it's really from your pituitary which is a gland, and different from your brain. Anyway, TSH is a loudspeaker that shouts, "Hey thyroid gland, can you start making more thyroid hormone?" and for most of you, your gland happily responds, "Yes!" and makes T4 (thyroxine) for you.

Now, as I've explained, T4 is a pro-hormone, it's completely inactive in the moment it's birthed from your thyroid gland. If your TSH is high, you can assume your tissue thyroid levels are low because your brain always gets the most thyroid. Now, if your TSH is normal, your test is irrelevant because your cells may still be starving even while your brain is getting some. You need to look at other tests. If there's one thing I want you to learn from my book it is this: The TSH hormone is really good for evaluating brain levels of thyroid hormone, it does not say much about tissue (cellular) levels of hormone. Your TSH level is blind to what's going on inside your cell and so TSH is not useful at finding people who are thyroid sick, that's why you may have fallen through the cracks.

TPO or Thyroid Peroxidase Enzyme. When your thyroid gland makes thyroxine in response to TSH shouting at it, the production happens with the help of this TPO enzyme. TPO is not a bad thing, it's a great thing but you often hear TPO cast in a negative light. The reason is that antibodies (the 'soldiers' in your body) can form against TPO enzyme, and that's the bad part. The enzyme itself is innocent and if anything, helpful! The antibodies against it are what light your precious thyroid gland on fire. When doctors test you for antibodies to TPO enzyme, they are trying to find out if you have Hashimoto's disease. Read Chapter 16, *Hashimoto's Disease.*

T4 or Thyroxine. This is the form of thyroid hormone released from your thyroid gland. It's inactive and must be activated (converted) to something else (T3) in order for you to feel well. Think of T4 like you would a snack bar! You can tote that around in your purse or backpack anywhere you go. You only tear it open when you're hungry. That's the same thing with T4. It is something carried all around the body, but it isn't used by the cell until it gets unwrapped. T4 has a choice, it can go one of two directions. See Table 2 (image of T4, rT3 and T3).

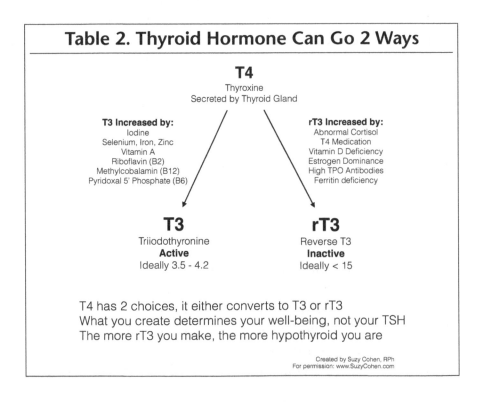

Table 2. Thyroid Hormone Can Go 2 Ways

T4
Thyroxine
Secreted by Thyroid Gland

T3 Increased by:
Iodine
Selenium, Iron, Zinc
Vitamin A
Riboflavin (B2)
Methylcobalamin (B12)
Pyridoxal 5' Phosphate (B6)

rT3 Increased by:
Abnormal Cortisol
T4 Medication
Vitamin D Deficiency
Estrogen Dominance
High TPO Antibodies
Ferritin deficiency

T3
Triiodothyronine
Active
Ideally 3.5 - 4.2

rT3
Reverse T3
Inactive
Ideally < 15

T4 has 2 choices, it either converts to T3 or rT3
What you create determines your well-being, not your TSH
The more rT3 you make, the more hypothyroid you are

Created by Suzy Cohen, RPh
For permission: www.SuzyCohen.com

In order to be activated to T3, it has to drop one atom of iodine, and it uses an enzyme. T4 hormone is commonly measured in the blood stream by conventional doctors and it can be normal even when you are thyroid sick. I don't want you to be dismissed again. I need you to learn, and teach your own doctor if you have to that T4 is not necessarily converted to T3 inside the cell. Therefore, levels of T4 are not useful to measure thyroid activity. T4 isn't always transported into the cell, or activated and so measuring it is fine, but only as part of a bigger thyroid profile. In people with chronic stress and depression, T4 will be normal, or sometimes high! You could be told you're hyperthyroid (too much), but that is a possible misdiagnosis due to the fact that T4 may not be transported properly into the cell, or converted to T3.

This is very very common if you've been ill for a few years. It goes back to what I taught you in the beginning of this book, that your thyroid gland may pump enough hormone (T4) so you're not technically "hypothyroid" but you could very well be "thyroid sick" because the T4 isn't going inside your cell (the transport system is broke).

T3 or Triiodothyronine Hormone. This is the unwrapped snack bar that I referred to above. It's the active form of thyroid hormone. Honestly, T3 is your dream come true, it's the hormone you want in all of your cells. When you read about how good you feel when thyroid hormone is optimized, they are really referring to T3 form. T3 will warm you up, make you happy, give you energy, make your hair grow. Production of T3 is halted in the presence of inflammatory chemicals and stress as you will soon see in the next chapter. There are studies to show that T3 dilates your blood vessels so as much as I want you to take this, I also want you supervised, be very careful with your levels if you happen to be taking it as a medication (Cytomel, Compounded T3). If you have heart disease please be careful taking too much T3 because it could backfire.

Like any good thing, too much is bad. Conversion from T4 to T3 can slowed down by all sorts of things including imbalances of progesterone and estrogen, binding problems to the receptors on your cells, transport issues and nutritional deficiencies.

Reverse T3 or rT3. This is a mirror image of Free T3. Imagine your left and right hand, they are mirror images of each other. The rT3 is there as your check and balance. It clears out excess T4. Think about it, if you had nothing but T3 in your body you would be wound up tight, and toxic from all the T3 because it's a stimulating hormone. The check and balance is rT3 and the rT3 keeps things in balance. I never want you to think of rT3 as bad. That said, excessive amounts of it are bad! The more rT3 you have, the more you feel tired, depressed and "inactive." You see, the compound rT3 lowers thyroid activity.

Too much rT3 will cause you to be clinically thyroid sick. The value of rT3 is very important to your health but it's rare when a conventional physician volunteers to test you for this. When rT3 is measured, and found to be high, it's also telling you that thyroxine (T4) isn't going into the cell. It's common to see high rT3 and high T4 when you test yourself. Certain conditions like stress cause you to make more rT3.

Reverse T3 is high in hibernating bears, no joke! I've gotten countless emails from some of you saying "I could not get my physician to order this lab test for me." The reason there's such obstinance is that physicians are taught rT3 is an inactive metabolite (by-product in the body), and that it doesn't do anything and therefore they rarely measure it. But think about it, is it really inactive? I mean, it IS doing something! It's blocking your receptor site and preventing too much T3 from being transported into the cell (which is fine). The problem is that when levels of rT3 go up too high, it locks the doors to your cell. So high levels mean you are not thyroid healthy. It is extremely important to me that you measure your rT3 so please ask your physician to test this next time they do your complete thyroid profile. If you are really up against a rock and a hard place, and you want this test, buy it yourself. I've arranged an affiliate website for you in case you want to order a blood test without any hassle. You use the home collection kits (or a local lab if a blood draw is required) and after you get your results, you take them to your physician for interpretation. My page is *www.DirectLabs.com/SuzyCohen*. This next part could be huge for you, and the words are rarely, if ever spoken. But I'm not afraid to say it: If you have high levels of rT3 don't use T4 drugs because you'll tend to make even more rT3, thus making yourself worse. Remember that. If you have high levels of rT3 don't use T4 drugs because you'll generate more rT3, instead of the biologically active T3 which makes you lose weight, look beautiful and live the life you imagine.

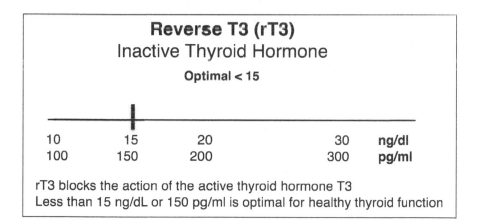

How to Lower rT3 Naturally

The following information could make a big difference for you and it may be all you need to do. Bringing down high levels of rT3 means that your cells get nourished with biologically active T3. These are some ways to lower rT3 naturally:

1. Increase selenium in your diet, or through supplementation.
2. Support your liver and consider a liver cleanse or supplements like milk thistle, glutathione or artichoke extract.
3. Reduce or eliminate drinking, smoking and refined foods
4. Switch from a pure T4 drug to a T3 medication. The T4 drugs (levothyroxine) tend to break down into more rT3 instead of bioactive T3.
5. Switch from natural desiccated thyroid to a T3 medication for awhile for the same reason as above.
6. Take adrenal supportive nutrients.

Enzymes Make the Magic Happen

If you have diabetes, fibromyalgia, depression, or you're over-weight, if you diet a lot, have leptin resistance, have high amounts of inflammation, or deal with a lot of stress you affect certain enzymes in your body that are responsible for thyroid hormone production and conversion at the cell level. This is a big problem.

Stick with me here, because understanding how your thyroid hormone gets activated (converted) in your body is important to you becoming thyroid healthy. Your precious human body has 3 different enzymes that push the gas pedal for you and make that wonderful T3 hormone happen!

I really dislike big words that are hard to pronounce but this one is important for you to know about. As a group these enzymes are known as "5′ deiodinase." The apostrophe symbol that you see after the number 5 is called "prime" so the whole thing is pronounced "5 prime dee-eye-o-denase." We have 3 different kinds of deiodinase enzymes and luckily, the scientists gave us a break and named them 1, 2 or 3 so they're abbreviated as D1, D2 or D3 and for simplicity, that's how I will refer to them from now on. D2 is specifically devoted to your brain, and it never leaves your brain.

Table 3. The "D" Enzymes
D1 converts T4 to T3 everywhere in your body except your brain
D2 converts T4 to T3 only in your brain
D3 converts T4 to rT3 all over your body except your brain
Your brain doesn't have D3 so it never makes rT3
The difference between D1 and D2 is that they antagonize each other. They both work to convert T4 to T3 but they are doing it in different parts of your human body. Think of them as working in opposing directions.

A Closer Look at the D Enzymes

I want to start at the top of your body (in your head), so I'm going to teach you about D2 enzyme right now.

D2 Enzyme. Converts T4 to T3 in the brain (and only your brain). Your pituitary gland sits at the base of your brain just in case you were daydreaming in high school biology about the football hunk you liked. Your pituitary has it's own local method for activating thyroid hormone. Just because you have adequate levels of T3 in your brain, doesn't mean anything about the rest of your body. This goes back to the difference between being hypothyroid and thyroid sick. Hypothyroid technically means your thyroid gland doesn't pump enough hormone out, whereas "thyroid sick" is my term for having enough hormone, but it doesn't get into your cells (tissues). My goal is to take you from feeling thyroid sick to feeling thyroid healthy!

There is a feedback loop with your thyroid gland. If you make too much T4, it signals back to the pituitary and says, "Stop making that TSH, we've got enough thyroid hormone now." TSH levels are dependent on T4 levels, not T3. You can have ALL the symptoms of low thyroid because you don't convert T4 into T3, but your T4 and TSH levels are perfectly normal. That sucks because you're not going to get treated correctly. When doc sees those "normal" thyroid levels on your lab test (or sometimes slightly elevated), you'll be handed a prescription for an antidepressant or fibromyalgia drug! Doctors miss people who are thyroid sick, by the millions so it's up to you to learn this distinction.

The most insidious part is that chronic illness confuses your lab results. When I say chronic illness, I am referring to various conditions, among them insulin resistance, diabetes, fibromyalgia, chronic fatigue syndrome, infections, chronic Lyme, depression, obesity, leptin resistance, high cholesterol or a chronic pain syndrome. If you have high inflammatory cytokines from any disease, or if you just deal with chronic stress, I am referring to you right now. I hope you're sitting down, I'm about to blow your mind again with something I learned the hard way on my own.

All these conditions have been shown to stimulate D2 and suppress D1 enzymes. The net result of this is that you get more T3 in your brain and less in the rest of your body. One more thing, these conditions stimulate D3 enzyme. If you recall, that converts T4 to the 'hibernation' form of thyroid called rT3 in the rest of the body, which then starves your cells for thyroid hormone. You are going to feel absolutely miserable, but your TSH and your T4 levels are likely going to be normal. You can refer to Table 3 The "D" Enzymes, if this is confusing. What's happening though, is that the cells in your body are now hypothyroid and your pituitary is actually a little bit "hyper" so it is sometimes slightly higher than normal on your lab test. Your TSH drops to normal and you'll be told you're fine. But the rest of your body is not getting the thyroid hormone it needs.

Fast forward to a few more years of suffering. Now more D2 enzyme gets stimulated which causes more T3 conversion in your brain (but not your body where you need it). So your pituitary gland senses plenty of thyroid hormone because it's gone up in your brain, while rest of the body and a trillion cells are starving for thyroid! The TSH will be normal though. See why the TSH test is useless in a person who is chronically ill? It's not measuring your tissue (intracellular levels) because it can't see inside the cell, it only knows what's happening in the brain, and up there, things look good. This is why I wrote this book, please help me spread the word about it. Not another day should go by without them knowing this precious information.

I understand you, I believe you, this miserable crappy state of affairs is not in your head, and if you're doctor dismisses you, take it as a cue to buy him a copy of my book. When we help one open-minded doctor, they help their patients all day long, hundreds each week, and it's a beautiful thing to have a trickle effect like that. If you have a physician that is not open-minded, I suggest you find another. Look on *www.FunctionalMedicine.org* for a Functional Medicine doctor. I'm not a doctor or I would help you myself, but I am a Functional Medicine practitioner (as a pharmacist). These docs think just like me and understand everything explained in my book. You'll be in good hands.

Chapter 3

Thyroid on Fire

You learned in Chapter 2 some pretty mind blowing stuff, particularly the part about how you are probably thyroid sick due to inaccurate interpretation of the TSH test, and reduced intracellular levels of thyroid hormone. And then you got to meet the family, and learn what each hormone does in your body. Isn't it just crazy how long-term illness can cause your test results to look in such a way that you're normal?! In other words, the longer you've been ill, the more likely you will have normal values on the standard thyroid blood test.

That was all explained in the previous chapter. Now, I want you to learn about the next puzzle piece. This kind of information is critical for you to speak intelligently to your doctor and request the tests you need to get healthy.

Thyroid disease is a predominantly female condition, approximately 8 women to 1 man. There are many discussions as to why this is. Some feel that women have fewer thyroid hormone receptors on the cell therefore less thyroid hormone can enter it. Some experts suspect it's because of hormone differences like the fact that women naturally make less testosterone, or that our estradiol and progesterone cycles slow down metabolism and increase fat storage.

As women, we are designed to carry more than one human being, meaning we can get pregnant! Immune cells sit poised and ready to attack anything other than our self, or our fetus. The theory is that this makes it easier for a woman to have an immune attack anywhere in the body, including the thyroid gland. If a family member has thyroid disease, your odds go up too. You're not quite as high risk if a female family member has it because that's fairly common but if a male has it then your risk goes up dramatically. Personally, I wouldn't pay attention to family risk too much, or genetics, since I believe both can be negotiated by your diet, vitamins/minerals, lifestyle and other factors within your control.

Thyroid Patterns

Thyroid hormone levels go up and down and change throughout the day. Secretion is pulsed not constant and it's aligned with your circadian rhythm, or your sleep-wake cycle. This means that hormone levels mirror your cortisol metabolism, with a TSH surge between 2 and 4 am. Remember, TSH is like a loudspeaker and in the wee hours of the morning, it shouts to your thyroid gland, "Sheesh, wake up you lazy thing, start making thyroid hormone!" causing the biggest release of thyroxine in the morning. The conversion of thyroxine to an active form of thyroid hormone goes on throughout the day and it happens inside your cells, out in your periphery, meaning everywhere but your thyroid gland.

There's no monthly rhythm for what the thyroid hormone does in your body but your monthly cycle affects activity. In a menstruating woman, estradiol, a form of estrogen you make, happens to increase 'thyroid binding globulin' and that lowers the efficacy of thyroid hormone, so right before ovulation and a week before menstruation, there's a point at which it's normal to feel more fatigued than usual, more irritable or foggy. These changes in thyroid hormone occur due to the higher circulating levels of estradiol. Unfortunately, the medications used for premenstrual syndrome or PMDD as it's called, are SSRI antidepressants (Prozac, Sarafem, Paxil, Celexa, Zoloft) and they do nothing to control the estradiol and even less to enhance your thyroid hormone! I'm wondering if you're taking the best drug for your needs. You may feel better on one week of natural thyroid hormone each month before your period rather than antidepressant drugs. Talk to your doctor.

Are You on Fire?

Here comes more mind blowing information: Thyroid disease is a problem of inflammation. It doesn't matter to me whether you are hypothyroid (gland doesn't produces enough hormone), or you are thyroid sick (you have enough hormone but you can't activate it in the cell), there is inflammation in your body. This is a biggie in terms of getting you well, so we have to talk about it, much as I dislike getting into science. Your body makes inflammatory chemicals, compliments of a pathway called NFκB, pronounced, "NF kappa B" and it stands for Nuclear Factor Kappa B. These inflammatory pain-causing chemicals are known more scientifically as "cytokines." You can think of these pro-inflammatory cytokines as sparks because they cause a smoldering little fire in your glands and tissues.

Why would your body go and do something mean like that? Why would it make all these chemicals that cause pain and inflammation? Because your body gets exposed to something it dislikes, or has an allergic reaction to something, that's why the inflammatory chemicals get sparked. Imagine your body dealing with stressors of all sorts, and being constantly inflamed (on fire) from your diet, your medications (they are chemicals you know), pollutants in the air from dry cleaning and carpeting, and toxic relationships for that matter. So many things can inflame your poor butterfly thyroid gland, essentially lighting your thyroid on fire! This situation is usually diagnosed as an autoimmune thyroid disorder, either Graves' disease or Hashimoto's (Chapters 10 and 17, respectively).

Whether or not you have been diagnosed with autoimmune thyroid disease is irrelevant to my discussion. What I am saying is that your thyroid gland is still "on fire" from cytokines, so please keep reading.

When this inflammation occurs, it occurs full-body, and it suppresses a system in your body called the Hypothalamus-Pituitary-Thyroid axis, shortened to "HPT axis." The net result of this is you feel tired, depressed, overwhelmed and frazzled; you hold on to weight, you cry easily, and your hair comes out in clumps when you brush it. Your periods become heavy or you have miscarriages, you get dry skin and fluid retention and you feel cold all the time ... see where I'm going with this? Systemic inflammation and high levels of cytokines (what I call thyroid bombs) cause adrenal dysfunction and many symptoms of thyroid disease. See Table 4 Thyroid Bombs. The catch here is that your TSH lab test may be perfectly normal (< 5 based upon standard testing) and you may be dismissed with "fibromyalgia" instead of what is really happening: Adrenal dysfunction with thyroid resistance. Most people feel better when their TSH is around 1.0, which is much different than what the standard reference range is on those lab tests.

Thyroid Healthy Tip

+ Do you feel better after you exercise? That probably means low thyroid.
+ Do you feel worse with exercise? That's usually a sign of poor adrenal function. You have to nourish and correct adrenal function before taking your thyroid, or while you take it. The thyroid doesn't heal until the adrenals are working better.

There was a study that showed a shot of one type of pain-causing cytokine reduced blood levels of free T4, Free T3 and TRH (Thyrotropin-releasing hormone) for a solid 5 days! There was a study that showed as your C reactive protein (CRP) went up, your conversion of T4 to T3 went down. In other words, this inflammatory chemical caused reduced transport and conversion of thyroid hormone.

Long story short, your goal is to reduce inflammation, not create it. There are many ways to do this. For example, you can eat fresh, organic foods and anti-inflammatory spices (turmeric for example), while eliminating some thyroid bombs.

Table 4. Thyroid Bombs
The following increase inflammatory pain-causing cytokines:
Grains, not just gluten, all of them Processed junk food Artificial sweeteners and colors Tap water contaminants Vegetable oil Plasticizers (drinking from bottled water) Dairy, more specifically casein, the protein in dairy Soy and soybean 'foods' Undiagnosed infections (H. pylori, Lyme disease, parasites, strep and others) Exercising vigorously Imbalanced hormones Cigarette smoking Alcohol Fluoride Most white breads (because of the additive bromine)

Flu Season Setback

It's like Murphy's Law, just when you are making some progress, November rolls around and you get sick. Most people come out of the flu just fine, but if you have thyroid disease, it goes without saying you have lowered immunity so the flu can knock you down. It's even harder to recover if you have adrenal fatigue too. If you are worried about flu season this year, I have a solution for you, Flunada spray. I love my solution, because it worked so well for me last year when I used it. Now, I serve as their Clinical Consultant. It's a non-prescription homeopathic throat and nasal spray formulated to provide relief from cold and flu-like symptoms. You spray it directly to your throat and nasal pathways, where most viruses enter the body. I like this product because it's natural, and the homeopathic blend is derived from eucalyptus, menthol and elderberry. It also has very solid laboratory testing data against both influenza and common cold viruses. This product is sold at drugstores nationwide and online. Visit *www.Flunada.com* for more information.

Are You Putting the Fire Out?

Thyroid medicines do not reduce inflammation, so they don't put the fire out. Here's a scary fact, no thyroid medicine addresses inflammation. Not even levothyroxine you ask? It's a top selling drug, but the answer is no, it is not an anti-inflammatory. It provides your body with bio-identical thyroxine (T4) that's all. Even Cytomel, the prescription drug that is bio-identical to T3 hormone, doesn't reduce inflammation. Synthroid and Cytomel are taken to simply raise your body's levels of T4 or T3 hormone, respectively. Sometimes you can take those two together, that is totally fine if your doctor suggests it. I'm not saying any of these drugs are bad, or good. I'm not saying to stop your drugs, I'm just pointing out their limitation, they do not reduce pro-inflammatory cytokines (they don't put the spark out). People react differently to medications and we all have an individual response. This is why it is imperative that you speak to your physician about your medication treatment and any supplements you would like to take. Some supplements that put the fire out include curcumin, vitamin D, probiotics and astaxanthin. These are all sold at health food stores nationwide.

Why Doesn't My Medication Work Anymore?

Dear Suzy, Why am I losing all my hair and feel cold and tired when I've been on levothyroxine for years? —Alice

Answer: Because your body isn't able to convert and use this drug which is pure T4. You are not able to convert it and use it in the cells.

The House Is Locked!

This is extremely important news. Inflammation not only hurts your adrenals and reduces T4 conversion, but it reduces the number of thyroid hormone receptors you have on your cells! Let's draw the analogy of each cell in your body to a house. You have trillions of cells, therefore trillions of houses. Each cell (house) has a receptor for thyroid hormone. Your stored inactive thyroid hormone (T4 or "thyroxine") has to be transported into the cell (remember MOST conversion of T4 to T3 is done inside the cell.) Let's zoom in and look at one house.

The house is dark, and it's locked up. The residents of this house are T3 (your active thyroid hormone). If your T4 hormone can't get inside this dark, locked house, it can't convert it to T3, and therefore it can't turn the lights on inside, turn on the heater and clean up the house. In real life that translates to you holding on to fat, losing brain power, developing heart disease, and feeling tired and cold.

What I'm saying is you can have perfect levels of thyroid hormone circulating in your bloodstream (labs for T4 and TSH will be normal), but it's locked out of the house! The transporter mechanisms aren't working to shuttle T4 in, or you have too much rT3 blocking the receptor so circulating hormone can't get in either! You could have halogens (chloride, fluoride, bromide) or other toxins blocking the cells (locking the house). Now, multiply this dilemma by trillions of cells, good grief right?!

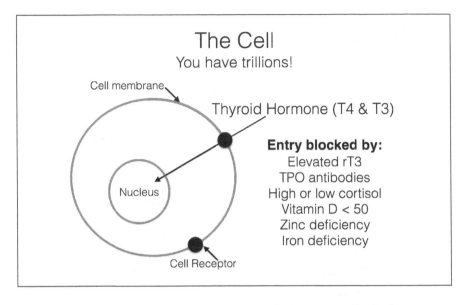

The Cell
You have trillions!

Cell membrane

Thyroid Hormone (T4 & T3)

Entry blocked by:
Elevated rT3
TPO antibodies
High or low cortisol
Vitamin D < 50
Zinc deficiency
Iron deficiency

Nucleus

Cell Receptor

Remember, the house in my example is your cell, the hormone needs to get into the house to turn on the lights and the power and warm it up (and warm you up for that matter!) Feeling cold all the time is a hallmark sign of hypothyroidism.

Inflammatory cytokines reduce the number and sensitivity of thyroid hormone receptors on the cell, this means the thyroid hormone cannot latch onto the cell and slip inside! The T4 cannot find the darn key to get inside the house! If you reduce inflammation in your body, the T4 finds the key, slips inside the cell and converts into T3, which is the equivalent of hitting the fuse box, which turns on the power. You feel fantastic! If you do not reduce inflammation, it does not matter how much thyroid medication you take, your cells can't use it. If you take T4 medications (like Synthroid, Levoxyl, Unithroid, Levothyroxine, and you have lots of inflammatory chemicals loose in your body, these T4 drugs don't work very well for you, since you cannot convert them to T3. They can't get in the house. Refer to Table 4 to see what Thyroid Bombs affect you. Also refer to Table 5 for the list of Medications Interfere with Conversion.

Would You Go to the Mall and Just Sit in the Car?

At some point, in order for you to feel thyroid healthy, T4 must leave your blood and cross your cell membrane to get inside your cell, where it's converted to T3. The point I'm making is that thyroid hormone is not diffused into cells, there is actually a transport system that is very active, shuttling hormone in and out all day. What if the thyroid hormone is not crossing into the cell? You could be the "poster child" for hypothyroidism if your transport system isn't functional. You want thyroid hormone INSIDE the cell, not outside. So that T4 value on your lab report isn't a clear picture, because there's no guarantee it's transported intracellularly. It's the equivalent of your husband taking you to the mall and saying you can have a gift, "Pick something out sweetheart." But when you get to the mall, you're just standing there, staring inside because the doors to the mall are locked. I can't tell you how I got that analogy, but it makes sense to me ;-)

Table 5. Medications Interfere with Conversion

Some drugs put a stop sign in front of T4 and prevent its conversion to T3. Among the most common offenders are:

- ✓ Beta blockers
- ✓ Chemotherapy
- ✓ Oral contraceptives (pills, patches, shots, etc)
- ✓ Menopause drugs, also termed HRT for "hormone replacement therapy"
- ✓ Lithium
- ✓ Anticonvulsants
- ✓ Corticosteroids (prednisone, hydrocortisone, etc)
- ✓ Theophylline

Do not stop taking those medications, some of them are needed for potentially life-threatening conditions like asthma or seizures.

Beam Me Up, Scotty!

Your thyroid activity is, in a sense, a two-step operation where transport and activation both have to take place. All of us Star Trek fans remember William Shatner saying that to his chief engineer Scotty. In order for Captain Kirk to materialize in the Starship Enterprise, he needed a transporter. The same thing is needed for thyroxine (T4) to cross over into your cells.

It's still being taught in some medical schools that thyroid hormone gets across the cell membrane by passive diffusion going from a place of higher concentration, to inside the cell where there's lower concentration. Can you believe that? But this is not true! Don't let anyone tell you that. Transport of thyroid hormone requires a specific transporter protein, and there are several:

Monocarboxylate transporter	MCT8
Monocarboxylate transporter	MCT10
Organic anion-transporting polypeptide	OATP1C1

I promise you, it's not passive diffusion, look at more than 40 references I've included in this book, and you will bang your head like I am right now. Doctors coming out of medical school today are going to assume this old-thinking unless we do something. Help me to heal others by getting this book in the hands of all of your friends. We are grassroots right now.

One of the most effective transporters is "monocarboxylate transporter 8" or MCT8, and the gene for this is on the X chromosome, so let's hope your mama had it. Genetic problems in any of these transporter systems in your body will cause clinical hypothyroidism, something I've been calling "thyroid sick" in my book. It causes higher levels of Free T3, which may lead your doctor into thinking that you are hyperthyroid, but that is not the case here. It just means your T3 is locked outside "the house" or rather your cells. Your lab tests reveal elevated serum T3 due to poor transportation into the cell, which could cause your doctor to tell you that you're fine, when you are not.

What can you do? Eat more mineral-rich foods, especially selenium, relax more. Cortisol shuts down thyroid activity, so avoid stress to bring it down, laugh more because it raises endorphins, and optimize your vitamin D levels. All of these will contribute to better transport. The number one thing you can do is to protect your cell membranes, and there is information on how to do that in Chapter 24, *Live Thyroid Healthy.*

Your Synthroid May Not Work Because of Transporter Issues!

Let me blow our mind right now and tell you that rT3 has the same exact transporter as your healthy, happy T3 hormone. Yep, that means the more rT3 you have, the busier the transporters are shuttling that over to the cell, but remember, it blocks your cells doorways and keeps the real deal (T3) from getting inside the cell! Darn it, that makes you thyroid sick, regardless of your TSH test (which I already taught you is a reflection of brain levels of thyroid hormone, it has nothing to do with cell levels of thyroid).

Now, let me warn you, if you take a blood test and you have high rT3, your Free T3 will come back elevated. Did they even check your rT3? Probably not, 90% of doctors will tell you I am crazy, and that you don't need to check it. Trust me, I'm going to get a lot of lip for telling you all of this (so please make it up to me, and leave me a 5 star review on Amazon!) Anyway, when you have high levels of rT3 in your blood, it's happening because of these transport issues, it's probably going to make your T4 high, and whatever T3 is circulating too. In this situation, T4 drugs like levothryoxine won't serve you well because they will just create more rT3 for you. These drugs preferentially form more rT3 than they do T3 in people with transport issues. In this case, Cytomel or Compounded T3 would be good, either along with your Synthroid, or instead of it. Proper testing will help your doctor to decide what to do, and it's a moving target! Your levels and labs change quite a bit, until you eventually find your groove.

In this situation I've described (poor transport of T4 and T3 into the cell), there's a completely different thing happening in the pituitary. Your pituitary gland has completely different transporters, so it is getting its thyroid hormone while the rest of your body is not. Your brain will not starve for thyroid, it has it's own devoted transporter and enzyme system, this is why evaluating the TSH is irrelevant, the TSH is based upon your thyroid hormone in your brain. It's the transporters below your head (the ones that work in trillions of cells all over your body) that are the rate-limiting step and the ones you need to have completely functional to lose weight, look beautiful and enjoy your life. If these transporters go down, Scotty can't beam you up! Want to know what conditions mess with your transporters? If you have any of the conditions listed in Table 6 Conditions That Block Transport, you cannot (repeat cannot!) trust your TSH if it comes back in the "normal" reference range. I think you will benefit from T3 replacement (or T4/T3 at the very least).

Table 6. Conditions That Block Transport	
Aging	High triglyceride
Anxiety	Insulin resistance
Bipolar	Infections
Chronic Fatigue Syndrome	Inflammation
Diabetes	Lyme disease
Dieting	Migraines
Fibromyalgia	Obesity
High cholesterol	Stress

Should You Avoid T4 Drugs?

The healthier you are, the more likely a T4 drug will work. T4 drugs don't have to be avoided, but they should also not be the gold standard of treatment for every single person. I think some combination of T4 and T3 might work better for the chronically ill, whether that combination is synthetic or glandular-derived is up to you. We're all unique. If you have any of the conditions in Table 6 Conditions That Block Transport, the T4 drugs don't work so great. Look at those conditions, some of them are really challenging disorders. Let me assure you that even slight reductions in cellular energy result in dramatic declines in T4 uptake (transportation inside the cell). This is the reason why T4 drugs don't work well in very ill folks. T3 uptake is less affected by those conditions. Your physician should test you properly.

My fear is (and it's happened a million times to many of you) is that when T4 is measured and higher than the normal reference range, you will be told that "your thyroid levels are within normal range so you're okay." You may be told, "Your thyroid is slightly high, not low, so this can't be a thyroid problem."

Stress alone will prevent a T4 drug from working optimally. You may find that your physician keeps upping your dosage (increasing risk of side effects) but you still feel bad, and you still feel thyroid sick and you're tired and melancholy and cold, with lots of muscle and joint pain and everything that goes with it. You feel like your thyroid medicine isn't working right?

Do you recognize yourself with what I have described? This is so common!!! That's why the key to getting thyroid healthy is to:

- ✓ Reduce inflammation in your thyroid gland
- ✓ Improve conversion of T4 to T3
- ✓ Reduce toxins and heavy metals that promote more rT3
- ✓ Improve transport of T3
- ✓ Protect your thyroid gland from gluten, casein and soy
- ✓ Protect your thyroid from fluoride, chloride and bromide

The answer is NOT to pump you full of more and more thyroid medicine. Supplements can help, however, most of the ones on the market today provide nutrients and co-factors or herbs that raise levels of T4, they don't improve conversion of it to T3, which is really what you want. If you are tested properly and you are T3 deficient, you have 3 medicinal ways to increase that T3:

1. Add a T3 drug to your current regimen of T4
2. Switch to a T4 and T3 combination drug
3. Discontinue the T4 drug for awhile and take only T3

The TSH test is the gold standard test for thyroid. The fact that it's used to determine if you're hypothyroid or not is the silliest thing ever! It's just one slice of the pie, and the least important. I'm saying, if your TSH is measured, who cares? I really don't care because the pituitary has it's own transport system which rarely fails. The pituitary gets what the pituitary wants, and it gets it first. The cells starve but the pituitary gets satisfaction. It's like your mom playing favorites and giving your sister all the good presents while you just watch. The TSH isn't a measurement of hormone in the cell. Your whole entire body could have low tissue T3, but the TSH often comes back normal. Scary huh? Does this explain why you feel so bad in the face of "perfect" or "normal" blood tests? You need adequate physiological amounts of T3 to wake you up.

Do Antidepressants Make Your Thyroid Work Better?

No amount of antidepressant will heal your thyroid gland, or make it work better. If you take T4 medication (like Synthroid, Levoxyl, Unithroid, Levothyroxine, etc), and are chronically ill, these T4 drugs don't work very well, since you cannot convert them to T3. If you recall, those inflammatory cytokines block your ability to convert T4 to T3, so you have more inactive thyroid hormone, than active in your body! You are a walking zombie. Antidepressants prolong the actions of various happy brain chemicals such as dopamine or serotonin, but they do not lift thyroid hormone. You can certainly take them together if you want to, but studies show thyroid hormone alone works better than some antidepressants in women.

It's A Fungus!

Did you know that yeast make their own neurotransmitters. Do you happen to get vaginal yeast infections? Do you have a white coating on your tongue, or have fungus on your nails? Even if you don't, you might still have an overgrowth of yeast in your body, or in your gut. Now, if you have anxiety to go along with the yeast, ask your doctor to do some genetic testing on you, or go buy a saliva test kit from 23andMe.com because it could be from a genetic problem with your COMT and/or MAO pathways. When these metabolic pathways are affected, you remain in a state of emotional anxiety due to the high excitatory chemicals. By that I mean high amounts of glutamate in your brain, and low amounts of GABA.

You have to negotiate this imbalance of brain hormones and resulting anxiety by reducing or killing off yeast, completely avoiding sugars and starches and taking supplements that reduce glutamate and raise GABA. Genetic testing can uncover the genetic portion, but you don't need to do that kind of testing to get well. For some of you, it can be as simple as changing your diet, and taking high-quality probiotics like Dr. Ohhira's brand for example. And you can tell over a few months if the feelings of anxiety come down. Lack of beneficial bacteria in the bowel can result in you losing 20% of your T3 thyroid hormone. Adrenal support is absolutely essential to this working, and for that you have many choices. I have seen good experience with simple herbs such as ashwagandha, by Organic India. Researched Nutritionals brand makes a new excellent formula called Energy Multi-Plex.

To support the production of GABA, I really like Honopure, a brand of magnolia brand extract made by Econugenics. This is a high quality product that is thought to improve brain hormones that relax you, such as GABA (the same hormone affected by Xanax for example). Honopure is natural, non-addictive and has other remarkable health benefits such as anticancer benefits. Drinking passionflower tea or taking liquid herbal extracts of it, can help with anxiety because it improves GABA.

Part II
Thyroid Testing

Chapter 4

Limitations of the TSH Test

The TSH test is a better screening test, and okay when done as part of a bigger thyroid profile test. The TSH range for what is "normal" is really not well correlated to what is "healthy." You see, when the powers-that-be figured out the "normal" reference range for the TSH test, they included lots of thyroid sick people in the group so the reference range is based upon sick people. When you match up with them, and you often will by the current standard, you will be told you are "normal" too. They should have only included healthy people who were full of vitality, after all that is who you want to emulate isn't it?

The TSH standard test only finds about 10%, perhaps 20% of people who are low in thyroid, the other 80% are dismissed as "heathy" or worse, misdiagnosed with a disease that is really a clue you have hypothyroidism, such as "depression." This is how most conventional clinicians treat your thyroid disease:

- ✓ TSH is high, give more thyroid medicine.
- ✓ TSH is low, give less thyroid medicine.
- ✓ TSH is normal, no need for treatment.

OMG! It's not that easy! Misdiagnosing thyroid disease is a medical disaster. Evaluating the TSH is the absolute *worst* place to evaluate your true thyroid status! Using this test means up to 80%

of people with hypothyroidism fall through the cracks. The TSH test is especially misguiding if you have any autoimmune disease including Lupus, Hashimoto's, Graves' or multiple sclerosis. It's apt to be inaccurate if you have insulin resistance, depression, live with pressure and stress, have high cholesterol or have any inflammation. Everyone has some type of inflammation in their body, we just live in that day and age.

You'll be prescribed some antidepressant which helps temporarily but over a few months you start to feel bad again. Why? Because antidepressant drugs don't correct thyroid hormone. People who take anti-depressants, suppress their own ability to create serotonin. Getting diagnosed correctly is key to getting well. It's Step 1 which is "S" for See a good doctor! More in Chapter 24, *Live Thyroid Healthy.*

Thyroxine is secreted from your thyroid gland which spreads throughout your body and once converted (activated) to T3 ultimately tells your tissues and organs how to behave nicely. The T3 regulates how fast your heart should beat for example and how fast you should burn fat.

The process can go awry for many reasons and cause you to feel like you're sick, or dying. The biggest tragedy in this country is the testing. You see, the gold standard blood test, called the "TSH Test" is what virtually all doctors use to evaluate thyroid hormone levels. This blood test almost always comes back in the "normal" range (about 80% of the time) at which point, your doctor says to you that nothing is wrong, when things in your body are horribly wrong.

The reason it has limitations is because it is not a measure of actual thyroid hormone, it's a pituitary hormone. TSH reference ranges differ depending on the lab, and how it's interpreted by your doctor. TSH is okay to use if you live 'off the grid' and you're healthy and enjoying your life with several million in your bank account and a perfect happy family. Is there anyone like this? If there is, her thyroid is probably perfect.

The more stressed and ill you become, the less reliable the TSH is. It's a blood test that should be considered a screening test, however, it is sadly used to diagnose thyroid disease, and gauge medication dosage. Big mistakes can occur relying on this blood test. Unfortunately, a lot of old-school conventional doctors won't treat you unless your TSH goes up above 4 or 5. What a medical catastrophe for you. I asked my good friend and colleague, Dr. David Brownstein about this. He is a medical doctor specializing in thyroid illness. He has written 12 national best-selling books, including *Overcoming Thyroid Disorders*. He and I hosted the *TheThyroidSummit.com* in 2014. Dr. Brownstein had this to share, "I have been treating thyroid patients for over twenty years. I can assure you that the proper diagnosis of a thyroid condition requires a thorough history, physical examination, basal body temperature measurements and a complete thyroid laboratory workup. The TSH test is one measure of thyroid function, but it certainly should not be used as the only indicator to determine if someone is suffering from a thyroid condition." For more information on this remarkable physician and his easy-to-read books (of which I have every one in my library!) visit, *www.DrBrownstein.com*.

If you were my best friend, I'd suggest you try to get your TSH levels between 0.1-1.0 and if it's above 1.0 or even 1.5 then ask for a trial course in medication. You should feel better, assuming your adrenals are in good shape. What I'm saying is that if your TSH is above 1.0, you have some degree of thyroid disease and may benefit from medication and lifestyle/diet interventions but really, the clinical picture is best. How do you feel? If you feel vibrant and happy and healthy with your TSH level (whatever it is) then you don't need treatment. The way you feel is very individual, and based on other parameters such as neurotransmitters, hormones and ferritin levels so treat yourself, not your blood tests.

This is straight out of the *British Medical Journal*, TSH is a poor measure for estimating the clinical and metabolic severity of primary overt thyroid failure. "In contrast to the good correlations with both circulating thyroid hormones, we found no correlation or only weak correlations with serum TSH."

Seniors might just have a slightly elevated TSH and be okay. As you get older, your TSH climbs a little bit, and that's okay, that's normal in fact. A study found that just under 7% of people 60 to 79 years old, and 12.5% of those aged 80 years or older have mild TSH elevations but do not require aggressive thyroid hormone replacement medication.

Chapter 5

The Best Lab Tests

You will get "thyroid healthy" much faster if you test your thyroid levels correctly. Many doctors mistakenly measure TSH and base your thyroid status (and drug dose) on this TSH. A new study from the *Journal of Clinical Endocrinology and Metabolism* finds your risk of death goes up (if hospitalized) if your T3 is low because your body is weakened. You can measure free and total T3 by yourself, order the kit through my link directly (or call them): *www.DirectLabs.com/SuzyCohen*. I've made this page to take the hassle out of testing for you. You can also ask your physician to order any test you find in my book. This chapter is devoted to helping you sort out what tests you should take, and what the numbers mean. There are structure and function tests, it's two pronged.

The Best Structure Test

The best structure test is an ultrasound, and I like it because it's safe, inexpensive and there's no radiation involved. An ultrasound is non-invasive (no needles or probing, yay!) and it creates images of your thyroid gland by bouncing sound waves off it. This can detect enlargement or inflammation of the gland but doctors don't utilize it as often as they should. I recommend this imaging study as part of your baseline workup. Any physician can order an ultrasound for you. No special preparations are needed.

The Best Function Tests

Free T4 or Free Thyroxine

Suggested Level 0.8–1.8 ng/dl

This is great to measure as part of a bigger profile, but it's not a good marker of your thyroid health all by itself. The reason is because it is energy dependent, and if your transporters are down, T4 is locked out of the cell and this number goes up (even when you feel bad). T4 can be hitched up to a protein, in which case it is no longer "free." Free T4 will go up especially if you have chronic stress, fibromyalgia or depression because the transporters that normally take it into your cell where you want it, go on break!

Total T4 or Total Thyroxine

Suggested Level 140–175 ng/dl

This value on your lab is the sum of both Free T4 and protein-bound T4 (hitched up T4). You'll often see this number on your standard blood tests and it's fine, but it's seldom of any value because what matters is your "Free" T4 (which is the T4 that is NOT hitched up to a protein).

Free T3 or Free Triiodothyronine

Suggested Level 3.5 to 4.3 pg/ml

This is one value that I insist you get. This is the amount of T3 that is not bound to a protein, so it's the form that is readily available to power up your cells and make you thyroid healthy. This is one of the best ways to evaluate your thyroid status. If you take a T3 medication (for example compounded T3 or Cytomel) don't take it the morning of your blood test.

Reverse T3 or rT3

Suggested Level < 15 ng/dl (also expressed as < 150)

I love this test for you! You will have to ask for it (perhaps even nag for it) or buy it directly from my lab page, *www.DirectLabs.*

com/SuzyCohen I would like to see this less than 150. The reason it's so important is because the more rT3 you have, the less of your 'feel-good' hormone (T3) gets into the cell. Some data suggests that reverse T3 decreases the absorption of T3 into the cell by 34%.

Free T3 to rT3 Ratio

Suggested Level > 2

This is the absolute best method to evaluate what's happening inside your cell. The ratio of 2 biomarkers has been discussed in highly respected medical journals, and there are resources dating back more than 20 years so this isn't something newly invented. I only tell you this because you may hear that this ratio is "meaningless." Trust me, it's not. It helps you understand tissue levels. You need both tests, and then you take the ratio of the Free T3 to rT3. It will evaluate tissue levels and you want this ratio to be greater than 2, preferably between 10 to 20. If the ratio is less than 2, you are thyroid sick.

Do you hate math? I'm so sorry but you have to do this division problem in order to figure out your ratio. The hardest part is getting your lab values to match in units. It was a nightmare for me to get my ratio the first time, it took me about an hour before I could get it because my tests use different measurements for each of those 2 biomarkers. The numbers have to be in the same "units" or the ratio is incorrect. For example, the same lab calculated my Free T3 in pg/ml (picograms per milliliter) but the rT3 was noted as ng/dl (nanograms per deciliter). That's 4 different units! Some labs measure things in pmol/l (picomoles per liter), further confusing it. You cannot request your measurement to be calculated the way YOU want it, you have to convert the units that they present you on your lab work. Unless you're a math whiz, this creates a kink in calculating your ratio of Free T3 to rT3. I've made it very easy for you by uploading a conversion tool that automatically converts your numbers to the correct ones, using a drop down menu. In about 10 seconds, you will have your ratio.

I've named it "Easy Thyroid Lab Converter" and it's posted at both of my websites, *www.ScriptEssentials.com/ThyroidConverter* and *www.SuzyCohen.com/ThyroidConverter*

Thyroid Healthy Levels

These are optimal measurements, and do not necessarily reflect the current standard of care "normals."

rT3	< 15 ng/dl (also expressed as < 150)
Ferritin	70–90 mg/dl
TSH	.1 to 1.5 mIU/l
Free T3	3.5 to 4.3 pg/ml
Total T3	140–175 ng/dl
Free T4	0.8–1.8 ng/dl

TPO antibodies less than 20 IU/ml
Free T3/rT3 ratio should be >2

Thyroflex Thyroid Test

It's super easy, and non-invasive so no blood samples are needed. Your physician can evaluate the reflex on your arm. Easy and affordable! Basically, he taps a muscle on your arm with a little reflex hammer (not a real one guys!) to see how the wrist and fingers respond. You have to hit the correct area, the brachioradialis muscle and a computer shows your response because you are wearing a sensor. This test has an extremely high sensitivity if it's done correctly. It offers an instant result, and if there's a sluggish reflex it's a slam dunk for low thyroid. Some doctors estimate that it works 90% of the time. I've asked practicing physicians about this test, and the consensus is the same: It's a better indicator of thyroid status than TSH because the "relaxation phase" of the test correlates better with your tissue T3 levels than a TSH blood test.

Simple Temperature Test

Suggested Temperature > 97.8

A classic test for thyroid disease is the basal body temperature test. Some people think it's old-fashioned and maybe it has been around a long time but I like this test because it's so simple, and there are no needles or blood involved. You simply take your temperature. If you are a a woman, your internal basal body temperature can fluctuate based on the day of your cycle. It can be lower or higher than normal this is why tracking your temperature during the month lends excellent clues. Check your temperature before days 19 through 22 of your monthly cycle, and remember Day 1 is the first day of bleeding for your cycle. Temperatures tend to lower as we get older, so keep that in mind.

To take your basal body temperature you just need to use the right thermometer. Buy one that is a basal thermometer, these are often sold to women seeking pregnancy because they can track ovulation based upon temperature. Such brands include "3M Nexcare," "Clearblue" or "BD" and they're sold at pharmacies and discount department stores like Target. Here are the directions to follow:

1. When you wake up in the morning, put the basal body thermometer under your arm before getting out of bed (within 5 min of waking up)
2. Thermometer beeps when done, usually after a minute
3. Temperature should be between 97.8–98.2 (considered normal)

If it's less than 97.8, your thyroid is not working efficiently and you're hypothyroid. If you are still menstruating, do it while you are on your cycle. Adult women (not menstruating) and men can do it anytime. Some people put the thermometer under their tongue (instead of their armpit). If you do that, then a normal temperature would be 98.8–99.2 degrees. An oral temperature below 98.8 is a strong indicator that you're thyroid sick. We all know that a cold body temperature goes with hypothyroidism right? But surprise, surprise, it doesn't always! What if your temperature is normal, but you still have hypothyroid symptoms? That can happen, it is sometimes a clue that you have antibodies attacking your thyroid (as in Hashimoto's or Graves' disease). I would do one blood test to evaluate your TPO and Antithyroglobulin antibodies, but I'd do it two times, using two different labs, and wake up early, you must get to the lab between 7 and 9 am when your antibody production is at its highest.

Be careful by going just by body temperature. Chronic illness will lower mitochondrial function (your 'mito' make the energy for your body) and they are little motors in your cell that generate heat and energy molecules (ATP). If those mito are dysfunctional (misbehaving), you'll be thyroid sick because of the poor transport of T3 into the cell. You may not know this but there's a popular assumption that way back, eons ago, the mitochondria formed a symbiotic relationship with humans. The mitochondria were a bacteria as we were evolving and decided that they worked better together, and instead of producing 2 molecules of ATP from a mito, we can make 38, and we have trillions of mitochondria (motors). The total weight of these mito is about 3 and a half pounds. You will not heal unless you support mitochondrial health.

Now, if you keep giving thyroid hormone based upon temperature, and it doesn't go up that is saying you probably have something else going on. It could be Lyme disease, which will also make your body temperature cold. Your doctor can determine what infection it is for you, it may not be Lyme, but the point is that undiagnosed infections will kill or maim your precious mitochondria, and that could be why you don't warm up to massive amounts of thyroid hormone. Guess what else makes you cold? Getting floxed, as in fluoroquinolone toxicity. These antibiotics act like chemotherapy in the body, and they are thought to poison your cells by splitting DNA strands. It's complicated, but when this occurs your body temperature may go down. So if you've taken quinolone antibiotics (ciprofloxacin, moxifloxacin, levafloxacin), and your temperature is low, then your thyroid medication dose will have to be adjusted upwards to account for this.

Take These Tests If You Have Chronic Fatigue

I offer solutions to help beat the fatigue in Chapter 23, *Solutions for Thyroid Symptoms*, but the underlying cause is often reduced ferritin (iron) and testing is important to uncover this. You may have a normal hematocrit, the standard test for iron but I'm telling you that your ferritin may be dreadfully low, despite the normal hematocrit.

Ferritin

Suggested Level: 70–90
This is a blood test. You can measure iron directly, or its storage form called "ferritin" to see the level. Evaluating ferritin was how I found out that my own thyroid hormone was low because my iron and hematocrit levels happened to be normal. Iron deficiency anemia is a condition resulting from too little iron in the body and is the most common nutritional deficiency in the world. The World Health Organization (WHO) estimates that 2 billion people (30%) of the world's population now are anemic as a result of iron deficiency. Left untreated, iron deficiency anemia can cause fatigue, headaches, concentration issues, irritability, dizziness, rapid heartbeat, brittle hair and nails, pica, and cold intolerance.

With low iron or ferritin you get reduced conversion of T4 to T3 or thyroid resistance, and there's less activation of thyroid in your cell. With low iron, it's usually assumed to be a problem with oxygenation. It's not so much a problem of oxygen carrying capacity, it's a problem of reduced thyroid activity. One snag though, if you happen to take iron supplements, you should not take those at the same time as your medication because it will partially inactivate your thyroid drug.

If you're cold quite often, it may be related to iron deficiency which happens to 20% of folks. Please read Chapter 14, *Iron Deficiency and Chronic Fatigue.*

Adrenal Hormone Test

When your thyroid activity goes down at the beginning of illness, your cortisol (adrenals) pick up the slack. Then eventually, they peter out. You may feel better initially on thyroid medicine, and then crash. This is likely because you have adrenal problems that have not been identified or corrected. The adrenal glands are fragile, and they control your body's inflammatory response, they secrete cortisol your stress hormone as well as aldosterone and epinephrine. If your adrenal glands are impaired, you become tired and hypoglycemic. I think most people who are thyroid sick, are also adrenally fatigued. In fact, I'm willing to bet almost everyone reading my book is adrenally worn out, as well as thyroid sick. This is not something most practitioners are willing to say, or test for.

We live in such a world where if you're low in thyroid, you're probably imbalanced in adrenal hormones (either way too high for your own good, or flat-lined 'undetectable' from years of stress). Low thyroid causes more adrenal function for awhile, until that crashes too, from extreme chronic stress. You have to ask what's broken, and why. Cortisol is an inflammation hormone. It's secreted from your adrenal glands. When you rest, the adrenals and thyroid regenerate, unless of course you have really crashed them, then you need adaptogenic herbs.

If you don't balance your adrenal hormones and nourish the adrenal glands first, you won't respond to the thyroid medicine. An automobile accident, childbirth, losing a loved one, or a bad break up can trigger years of adrenal problems. This creates a problem with thyroid. The two go hand in hand. Here's how you can tell. If you can't tolerate thyroid medicine, it's a sign you need to nourish the adrenal glands. If you keep having to raise your dosage, you have adrenal problems. If you don't respond well to thyroid medicine but you have all the symptoms, again, you have adrenal problems. You know you have adrenal problems if you start producing epinephrine instead of cortisol, and you can tell easily because you become more anxious than you've ever been. Almost everyone who has chronic fatigue or fibromyalgia has some degree of adrenal dysfunction. I offer some solutions in Chapter 23, *Solutions for Thyroid Symptoms*. You may also have progesterone deficiencies, or magnesium deficiencies, which tax your adrenal function. It just gets to be one big vicious circle, but the starting point for you to get "thyroid healthy" is with your adrenals.

Testing your adrenals is essential, especially if you have a poor response to thyroid medications. No amount of thyroid hormone will work if your adrenals are worn out. You must (repeat must) correct your adrenal imbalances before you drop a lot of thyroid hormone into your system. Some conditions like lots of stress, chronic infections, depression, fibromyalgia and chronic fatigue cause your brain to secrete a less bioactive TSH for the same level of TSH, so you have lower levels of T4 and T3.

Be careful not to overdose yourself on thyroid medications, you have to correct the adrenal dysfunction first, and then you'll have a better response to your thyroid medicine. A common mistake practitioners make is to keep raising the dose of thyroid medicine to get you to feel better, but I'm saying that you should correct the adrenal dysfunction first, then you will be more sensitive to the thyroid medicine, and you'll feel better from head to toe.

There are adaptogens that work well for adrenal support, such as ashwagandha, panax ginseng, rhodiola and others. Entire books are devoted to the subject of adrenal health so I'm not going to tackle that here.

The crucial information I'm sharing now is that adrenal dysfunction might need to be corrected in order for you to respond properly to your thyroid medicine, don't just keep upping the dose! Thyroid medicine is not like a controlled substance or pain medication. In other words, those drugs cause addiction, and tolerance and you need higher dosages to get the same effect. This is not the case with thyroid medicines, you don't get addicted or tolerant to any of them, so you should never need more from a physiological standpoint unless you're resistant. And you could be if your adrenals are worn out. Bottom line is if you're having to up your dose every few months, it's because your condition is declining, or you have underlying adrenal dysfunction that no one is taking care of.

Thyroid Antibodies

Suggested levels as follows:

> Thyrotropin Receptor Blocking Antibody < 1.75 IU/ml
> TSI Immunoglobulins < 130% used for Graves' or multi
>   nodular goiters.
> TPO (thyroperoxidase) Antibody should be < 30 IU/ml
> Thyroglobulin Antibody (TGAb) should be < 3 ng/ml
>   or < 40 IU/ml
> TSH stimulation blocking antibody (TSBAb) < 40%
> Thyroid Stimulating Antibody (TSAb) < 140%
> Thyrotropin Receptor Antibody (TSHR) gene

The tests above are blood tests that you might see on your lab, they are named various ways so I've listed all the names. These biomarkers could indicate autoimmune thyroid disease. The attack on your thyroid gland will basically eat away the gland so you want these antibodies to come back normal, or low. If they're above normal reference range, you need to strictly avoid soy, casein and gluten. In fact, avoid all grains and lectins completely.

T3 Uptake

Suggested Level 24–39%

This essentially measures the amount of proteins that tote T4 around in the blood. It's going to be inaccurate if thyroid binding globulin (TBG) is abnormal. I don't rely on this at all since results can alter based upon you taking medicine, or having medical conditions other than thyroid disease. If you take drugs that compete with endogenous T4 production (like levothyroxine for example), then this number could change. This isn't foolproof, but generally speaking the value of T3 uptake should be low if you are hypothyroid, and it should be high if you are hyperthyroid. It's mentioned in my book because I want to be complete, and you'll see it on your labs but it's not a good indicator of your status since it is affected by many factors.

Iodine

Suggested Level 100–199 µg/l

Everyone wants to know their iodine level and it's fine by me. The iodine is taken up by your thyroid gland which is a sponge for it. You need this mineral to manufacture thyroid hormone. If you're deficient in iodine, you will have low levels of T4. The best way to evaluate iodine is with a 24 hour urine catch. I'm not excited about the practitioners who use those skin tests. I think they will be positive on probably every single person so don't rely on it. Low iodine doesn't necessarily require high doses for a long term. You have to be careful not to take too much, just supplement or eat iodine-rich food until you're levels normalize. You could be iodine deficient if you take a drug mugger of iodine such as a fluorinated drug. See Table 9 "Could Your Fluorinated Drug Crash Your Thyroid?" which can be found in Chapter 8, *Thyroid Thieves Lurking Everywhere*.

Sex Hormone Binding Globulin or SHBG

Suggested Level Women < 70 and Men < 30

This is a blood test to evaluate SHBG. What does "sex hormone" have to do with thyroid hormone? A lot, at least in women. It doesn't correlate well in men though so I wouldn't track SHBG in men. This biomarker goes up in response to 3 things, estrogen, insulin or thyroid hormone. They correlate directly. If SHBG is low, it means one of three things. You either have:

1. Reduced estrogen
2. High levels of insulin (diabetes will follow)
3. Low thyroid hormone

The best place to start is to get a hormone level on the estrogen and I'd suggest a 24 hour urine evaluation. Evaluate estrogen levels and replace estrogen until you get a normal level. Then retake the SHBG blood test. If it's still low, that means you're low in thyroid hormone. If you take thyroid hormone and SHBG doesn't go up, it proves thyroid resistance, or what I've been calling thyroid sickness in my book.

The reference range differs but for our purposes, when I say "low" SHBG I mean less than 70 for a woman, and less than 30 for a man indicates you have either low estrogen or low thyroid (or possibly both). You could benefit from straight T3 (as opposed to combination hormones like T4/T3 drugs or straight T4 drugs. If I were a doctor instead of a pharmacist, and you were my patient, and you had high SHBG, I would tell you to lower your insulin first, before starting on thyroid medicine. I've written a comprehensive article on how to do that, and why it's so important. I've posted that article on my website, entitled, "Many Diseases Linked to High Insulin, The Longer Story." A serum insulin over 10 is trouble, and over 25 is a slam dunk for diabetes so I'd bring down insulin. My article will tell you how to do that using natural supplements such as quercetin, resveratrol and other nutrients. There's more about that whole subject in my diabetes book, *Diabetes without Drugs* (Rodale 2010).

Taking thyroid will definitely help to bring down SHBG, but reducing insulin will be better for you. It will allow whatever thyroid medicine you take to work better. Let's say you begin medicine for your thyroid. If you're taking oral thyroid medications, the medication will go through the liver first and make much higher T3 in the liver, so I want to warn you that if you measure SHBG and it's still low after a few months of taking thyroid medicine, it's a sign you're not getting enough thyroid. Your dosage should be adjusted upward by a practitioner who fully understands this and can supervise you. SHBG should increase when taking thyroid medication, so if it does not, that means you have thyroid resistance (thyroid sick); there are some nuances that your doctor will understand because your age has something to do with it too.

Leptin

Suggested Level < 12

This is a blood test. As you gain weight, you secrete more leptin from the fat cells. In a perfect world, it tells the brain we have enough stored fat so leptin reduces our appetite, and sends messages to help us burn fat. The problem is that most people have "leptin resistance" which means that no matter how much leptin you create from those fat cells, the brain doesn't see it. Not good. When your brain thinks your starving, you burn less calories, your appetite becomes voracious and every morsel of food you eat gets stored on your belly! Until you address leptin resistance, you're not going to lose weight. A leptin above 12 is not considered healthy, it's causing weight gain, aging you faster and increasing your risk of infertility, diabetes and heart attack. High leptin is associated with belly fat, cancers and type 2 diabetes. Leptin goes up if you take the drug dexamethasone, or insulin shots, and certain other hormones used for menopause. Leptin rises if you don't sleep well, and if you have any kind of perceived stress.

If you diet a lot, or exercise too intensely, this will lower your T3 levels, and increase rT3, but your TSH will be normal. The more you diet, the more you reduce your metabolism (the opposite of what you want) by about 25%. What does this mean? If you are having difficulty losing weight, you can check your leptin, you want it under 12. If it's above 12 this means you have low T3 levels (intracellular thyroid hormone) and higher rT3. If you have high leptin, and high rT3, the last medication I recommend for you is a T4 drug (levothyroxine), however, it's a mistake made every day, to millions of you! Don't go too low on your leptin, track it with blood tests. Very low levels are now thought to contribute to dementia or Alzheimer's.

Take These Tests if You Have High Blood Pressure or Heart Disease

HS CRP or "High Sensitivity" C Reactive Protein

Suggested Level < 1mg/L

A blood test. This is an inflammatory chemical that can help tease out whether or not your risk for heart disease is high. This is important because a fatal heart attack is possible with a clinically "normal" TSH in women. No joke! The study was published in 2008 in the *Archives of Internal Medicine* and the researchers made no bones about it, "The results indicate that relatively low but clinically normal thyroid function may increase the risk of fatal coronary heart disease." They were looking at TSH between 0.5 to 3.5. So evaluating your HS CRP gives you one a quick way to evaluate cardiac risk. You can lower this with B vitamins. Before you lower it though, you should ask yourself the question, "Why is my CRP high?" The most common cause is malabsorption of a few simple B vitamins needed to break the molecule down, things like folate and natural B12. Malabsorption is usually related to a leaky gut. Always ask why an inflammatory marker is high, it is almost always traced back to the bowel, most of us have inflamed bowels or leaky ones from years of insult. It's all fixable in time, with the help of digestive supporting nutrients and supplements like enzymes, probiotics, glutamine, aloe and others. This reminds me of why it's so crucial for you to take B vitamins that are "methylated" in their bioactive form. If you take regular B vitamins sold at deep discount retailers and chain pharmacies, you often get inactive pro-vitamins that don't work until your body activates them. That's a waste of your antioxidants and liver enzymes. Just pay up front a little more and get bioactive nutrients. For example, 5-MTHF (termed methylfolate or quatrefolic) is better than folic acid. Pyridoxal 5' phosphate works immediately, whereas pyridoxine doesn't, it has to be converted. It's essential to take bioactive nutrients to get optimal effects, don't rely on your body to do you any favors. Visit my online store if you ever want this *www.ScriptEssentials.com.*

Cholesterol Particle Size and Number

Suggested Level Varies, Refer to Your Test
I don't care much about your total cholesterol. In fact, checking total cholesterol and values for LDL and HDL is old school. It doesn't say anything about the particles or numbers of cholesterol. In this case, size does matter and you want it big. I'm not kidding here, the particle size of your LDL cholesterol is incredibly important, and this research is fairly new. The smaller your LDL particles are the worse it is. You see, there is a subset of LDL cholesterol and we've found that small dense LDL cholesterol is highly inflammatory and toxic to blood vessels.

We all want HDL high don't we? But certain HDL particles can be bad, did you know that? Again, you have to know the particle size and number, and the subfractions of these cholesterol particles. You can have this test done by Berkeley Labs, *www.bhlinc.com* and the name of the test is "Lipoprotein Subfractionation by Ion Mobility." If you're the person who is testing cholesterol, this is the test you should be taking, or an equivalent by another lab. The standard way cholesterol is tested is useless if you ask me. I'd save your money until you can take this type of test through Cleveland Heart Clinic, *www.ClevelandHeartlab.com.*

Are Your Muscles Wasting?

It could be low growth hormone or low testosterone, but it could also be thyroid problems. High rT3 levels could represent a catabolic state which is where your body is breaking down and you're losing muscle. Unless you are some type of athlete, purposely seeking a temporary state of catabolism, this condition is not something to welcome. For our purposes here, being in a catabolic state refers to an overall decline in health, sagging skin, atrophied muscles and weakness. It could be due to many things, including a rise in rT3. Reduce this biomarker with my tips on page 21.

Human Growth Hormone or HGH

Suggested Level 0.5–8 ng/24 Hours

Growth hormone levels are sometimes low in people with thyroid disease and even though it's unusual, when you find out about it (and replenish levels), it's fantastic because it speeds your healing process. In an adult, symptoms of low growth hormone may include reduced cardiac output, reduced left ventricular mass, loss of muscle mass, reduced exercise capacity, melancholy or depression, poor concentration, memory impairment, fatigue or weakness and sometimes social isolation. When you treat an adult with thyroid hormone, usually the growth hormone begins to balance and visa versa, if you give growth hormone, it improves conversion of T4 to T3. You can give both together (thyroid and growth hormone replacement). But how do you know if you need growth hormone? Consider your symptoms and various tests. In fact, there are many ways to determine the various growth factors in your body. Some people go by IGF-1 alone and others take a ratio. IGF-1 levels determine how fast you age.

Here's one of the best ways to determine your thyroid status and growth factor status. You take one blood test that evaluates two markers, then you take a ratio. I'm suggesting a ratio of IGF-1 to IGFBP3.

I know that's a lot of initials but I wouldn't reach this far and try so hard to help you if I didn't think it was worth it to you. It stands for the ratio of two important growth hormones in your body. More specifically this is the ratio of Insulin-like growth factor 1 (IGF-1) to Insulin-like growth factor binding protein 3 (IGFBP3). It causes shorter stature and poor growth. Thyroid hormone levels are associated with these growth factors. We knew way back in 2001 that hypothyroid patients have significantly lower ratios of this than healthy folks. What is interesting is that levothyroxine (a T4 drug) does not correct the ratio, but iodine does. Replenishing iodine helped increase IGF-1 and thus improve the ratio. Very high levels of IGF-1 as well as very low levels of IGF-1 are associated with cardiovascular risks. You want this growth hormone in the normal reference range. If it's very low, the ACE inhibitor drug class is known to increase levels. Popular ACE (Angiotensin Converting Enzyme) inhibitor drugs include lisinopril, enalapril and benazepril. To increase IGF-1 naturally, eliminate carbohydrates and sugar, go to bed on time (so you can produce growth hormones during deep sleep), and don't tax your liver. It's your liver that converts growth hormones to IGF-1. Now, if that IGF-1 is higher than normal, you should attempt intermittent fasting, because if you can go without food for about 12 hours, your body will start to repair it's DNA and IFG-1 will come down.

Take These Tests if You Have Anxiety, Depression or Insomnia

Discovering abnormalities in some other tests could be very telling for you, and why you are experiencing your plateful of symptoms. It's not just about the thyroid profile, it's about other labs that are just as important. You can do these one at a time if budgeting is an issue.

B12 and Folate Levels. If you have poor acid secretion in your gut (see above), you will likely have low levels of B12 and folate and this can lead to depression, cervical dysplasia, high homocysteine, nerve pain, fatigue, confusion and all sorts of other thyroid problems. It's a cheap test, I'd do it as part of your routine lab work. If you supplement, the correct, bioavailable forms are "methylcobalamin" for vitamin B12, and "5-MTHF" or "L-methylfolate" for the folate, NOT folic acid which I no longer recommend.

Vitamin D
Suggested Level above 50 ng/dl
This is a blood test. Vitamin D testing is important because it could uncover your Hashimoto's disease, and restoring levels could help you with any type of autoimmune disease. Not everyone can convert the 'sunshine vitamin' to an active form. In fact, there's a genetic mutation called "VDR BSM" that causes some of you to not be able to utilize your vitamin D very well. Genetic testing at 23andMe.com can uncover this. You see deficiencies of vitamin D in people with autoimmune disorders so I recommend the D test for everyone, because low levels could explain your thyroid disease, melancholy, chronic infections, heart palpitations, muscle aches or bone loss. I'd like to see this number above 50, closer to 70 might be in order for some of you too. The ratio of 2 different blood tests could be even better. You would take the following tests:

Vitamin D 1,25
Vitamin D 25
The ratio of those should be < 2

An example would be the following results:
Vitamin D 1,25 = 60
Vitamin D 25   = 20
$\frac{60}{20} = 3$

and that's greater than 2 so you don't need to supplement.

Neurotransmitter Tests. Your serotonin might be off causing you to crave sweets and coffee, anything to quickly feel good. It's a brain chemical involved in self-esteem, and happiness. Dopamine could be askew, this is your passion hormone, excess amounts cause irritability, while low levels cause tremors. The neurotransmitter adrenaline (a.k.a. epinephrine) is hindered in thyroid disease which is another difficult-to-tease out situation that causes depression, weight gain, low ambition, procrastination, fatigue and all sorts of mood imbalances. I think the best test for this is a urine analysis (not blood) and I recommend Neuro-Science labs for this kind of testing. You can ask your doctor to become a practitioner for them and order the test for you, but this could take a few weeks. You can also go to my lab page *www.DirectLabs.com/SuzyCohen* to directly buy this test, and other excellent tests to evaluate neurotransmitters. One of the best is the NeuroAdrenal profile.

Correcting neurotransmitter imbalances can go a long way in making your thyroid medicine work better, and making you feel better. It isn't really hard to do, please don't feel challenged by this whole concept. You pee in a container, and send it to a lab, they send your doctor back results in a couple of weeks. If your serotonin is low for example, a little (low dose) 5-HTP could help, and if it's high, a little riboflavin might work. If your dopamine is low, a little tyrosine or DLPA could help, or perhaps N-Acetyl Tyrosine and so on. These are just ideas, and you should be very careful with your brain hormones. I can't figure out what's right for you but I think you can with the help of a good doctor. Remember that seeing a good doctor is the first step in my "Script" to get you well. You can read more about the "Script" in Chapter 24, *Live Thyroid Healthy*.

Take These Tests If You Have Food Sensitivities or Digestion Problems

Gastrin. This is a digestive hormone you make which produces stomach acid. If you are hypothyroid or thyroid sick, the level is likely low.

When gastrin is high, it means that stomach acid is low so gastrin comes to the rescue and says "Stomach cells, please make stomach acid." Gastrin is important because it helps you to produce HCL, as in hydrochloric acid. You want some stomach acid. Gastrin is a hormone that responds to the amount of stomach acid present in your stomach. If there's not enough acid, gastrin will rise to stimulate acid production. If there's plenty of stomach acid, gastrin hormone goes down. Certain problems of course, like Zollinger-Ellison Syndrome will cause continuously high levels of excess acid, ulcers and loose bowels. High acid is easily treatable with acid blockers, but low acid is a problem for people with thyroid illness.

If your stomach acid levels are low, this is termed hypochlorhydria and it is very common in people with hypothyroidism. It's a new concept isn't it, to think about low stomach acid as opposed to high! If you watch TV for even 30 minutes, you're apt to see drug commercials convincing you that you have high stomach acid, so what I'm saying is probably a shock. I know there are so many antacids and acid blocking drugs to reduce your stomach acid, but I must convince you that you need some acid to become thyroid healthy. You will need HCL (yes, acid) to digest your meals, in order to extract nutrients and key minerals which support thyroid health. When you have enough acid in your gut, your gastrin hormone will go down to normal range.

Supplements of "Betaine HCl" or "Betaine with pepsin" could add acid to your digestive tract. You take them with food. How do you know if you need acid? You don't feel good when you eat meat. Your nails break easily, and you feel tired a lot. You need acid to absorb nutrients like iron, magnesium, copper, zinc, B12, folate and proteins so being hypochlorhydric means your body is starving for nutrition, regardless of what you eat. Stomach acid is necessary for your immune system. The acid from your stomach is a first line defense mechanism from the bacteria and other germs that enter your body. The acid literally helps prevent bacteria from colonizing and growing out of control.

Symptoms of low acid (hypochlorhydria) include burping, gas immediately after eating, bad breath, bloating, fatigue or heartburn. Correcting your acid levels by taking betaine with your meals can translate to higher energy levels, as well as better thyroid production. It works because betaine HCl increases your hydrochloric acid, which helps you digest your food and get all the nutrients out of it. It helps you get vitamin B12 from your food, particularly important if you have nerve pain (neuropathy).

Low acid in the gut could mean H. pylori infection, and that's not the only bug. In case you didn't realize, stomach acid is a huge component for our immune system and the acid "kills" some pathogenic bugs in your food. If you have a feel-full sensation very quickly while eating, it could be that your acid levels aren't high enough, and when that occurs your stomach delays emptying. This causes you to feel bloated, and feel full faster than normal. Determining a healthy betaine dosage is important. How do you figure that out? You take 1 capsule with your meal, and if there's no heartburn then take 2 capsules at your next meal. If you still don't feel 'the burn' then take 3 capsules at your next meal (or wait until tomorrow if you're nervous about it). The point is, when you feel the burn, you back off to the last dosage you took. It takes 4 capsules for me to feel the burn, so I usually take 3 (sometimes 2 capsules) with lunch and dinner. This treatment is something to discuss with your doctor because my gastrin levels were normal, yet I was still hypochlorhydric. Betaine would never be advised for someone taking antacids or an acid blocker, it is contraindicated in that case. Which leads me to another comment. People with so-called "heartburn" or "reflux" might be misdiagnosed anyway, and might be taking acid blockers when what they really need is more acid. Don't get me started, it's the makings of another 100 pages! For more on relief for gastric distress, I recommend my friend Martie Whitteken's book, "Natural Alternatives to Nexium, Maalox, Tagamet, Prilosec & Other Acid Blockers." Martie is a certified clinical nutritionist and a radio show host, and you can learn more about her at *www.RadioMartie.com*. Please also watch my YouTube videos on marshmallow root and slippery elm.

Gluten and Grain testing. The only lab I recommend for this is Cyrex because they check for all the different parts of the gluten molecule, and they test for the other grains that cross-react. I recommend Array #3 and Array #4 for you. This test is important for everyone with thyroid disease because I think a lot of you have autoimmune thyroid disease, and don't know it. Hashimoto's drives most cases of hypothyroidism. If you have this (or Graves' disease), you should think seriously about going grain-free and Cyrex testing can confirm for you if you have this food sensitivity. *www.CyrexLabs.com*.

Gliadin, the protein from gluten increases zonulin causing a leaky gut. Casein from dairy can too. These proteins lodge in your thyroid and cause inflammation. The less you eat of them the better. You can protect yourself from some of the assault by including gluten and casein digestive enzymes. One enzyme is called DPPIV and I put it in my unique formula, ThyroScript (*www.ScriptEssentials.com*). I read a lot in journals, and I go to many lectures and hear the almost frenzied discussion of gluten. No doubt! There are books written on the topic. I was a featured speaker for the world's first Gluten Summit, hosted by my friend Dr. Tom O'Bryan, a gluten expert. There's more to the story of gut inflammation than just gluten as we all learned. There's a particularly harsh lectin, called wheat germ agglutinin or WGA for short. It's present in our modern day wheat (Triticum aestivum) and highly problematic! It is implicated in many reactions that cause cell death and it causes your body to pump out tons and tons of inflammatory cytokines! People who eat "whole wheat" today think they are doing themselves a favor, but WGA is actually more concentrated in whole wheat because it's in the bran. This is why eating a grain-free diet can make you "thyroid healthy" much faster than you can imagine. Give it a try for 2 months, you have nothing to lose but weight, and everything to gain including your health.

Zonulin. You can measure this protein with a blood test. Zonulin is a protein that is elevated in people with autism, lupus and digestive diseases like Crohn's, Celiac and others. I recommend zonulin testing for people with thyroid disease, especially those who suspect Hashimoto's or Graves' disease. Zonulin is a substance that wedges a big space between the cells in your intestine. Basically it opens the door in your gut to cause "leaky gut" and all the microscopic food particles (mainly proteins) that would otherwise get digested, leak out into your bloodstream. Once that occurs, your immune cells get to work and chase down the invader. If the proteins that leaked out take up residence in your thyroid gland, you have an autoimmune disorder like Hashimoto's or Graves' disease. Your immune system goes crazy and churns out inflammatory pain-causing compounds (called cytokines) and as more damage occurs, your microvilli get flattened out. These are microscopic hairlike extensions of the cells in your gut. Think of a thick shag rug (microvilli) that gets picked clean and loses all the fuzziness, becoming a flat mat. That's how it occurs, and the big deal about that is you can no longer absorb nutrients from your food, or dietary supplements. That means your thyroid hormone production is compromised because you do not have the minerals and vitamins on board to make hormone. So measuring zonulin is important. Evaluating zonulin is critical if you have Celiac disease. You want the number to be low. When zonulin is high, you have bigger holes between the cells, and therefore a leakier gut. See Table 7 Reduce Zonulin, for supplements that can help.

Table 7. Reduce Zonulin

The best way to reduce zonulin is to remove the food allergens such as soy, gluten, casein, eggs or whatever you react to. You should also find out if you have gastrointestinal parasites, H. pylori or other offending pathogens. All of the following supplements may help you reduce zonulin:

- ✓ Diamine oxidase (DAO)
- ✓ Glutamine
- ✓ Hops
- ✓ Glycosaminoglycans
- ✓ Quercetin
- ✓ Immunoglobulins
- ✓ Probiotics

Chapter 6

5 Ways Your Doctor Misdiagnoses You

You could have all the symptoms of low thyroid and yet be misdiagnosed with depression, chronic fatigue syndrome or fibromyalgia. How can this tragedy happen? It's because they are evaluating you by the TSH test, and it will come back in the normal reference range, or possibly high, leading your doctor to suspect that you're thyroid function is normal, when it's anything but! Why would I say something that flies in the face today's standard of practice? Because you rely on me for the truth, isn't that why you buy all my books?! I don't parrot what everyone else is saying just to keep the peace. I'm here to help you. TSH testing may be every one else's gold standard test, but it's rust to me. It's only a marker for the pituitary levels of T3 and says nothing about your tissue levels. In fact, the more miserable you feel, the more apt your TSH comes back as normal! Yeah! Crazy isn't it?!

Numerous diseases cause an increase of pituitary T3 levels with reduced tissue T3 levels. The TSH doesn't pick up the fact that your cells are starving. Such conditions include stress, depression, insulin resistance and diabetes, aging, caloric restriction, chronic fatigue, fibromyalgia, obesity and exposure to toxins or plastic chemicals. This is all explained by my friend Dr. Kent Holtorf, a pioneer in the field of thyroid conditions and the medical director of Holtorf Medical Group, specializing in evidence-based therapies for hard-to-treat illnesses. He is one of my thyroid heroes. For more information on Dr. Holtorf, visit his non-profit site the National Academy of Hypothyroidism at *www.NAHypothyroidism.org.*

To get more clarity about what is happening inside your cell, and see if they are starving for thyroid, you can take the ratio of Free T3 and rT3 and see if it's > 2. Calculating the ratio of Free T3 to rT3 is kind of hard because labs use various units to express the values of those 2 biomarkers. I've made it very easy for you by uploading a conversion tool that automatically converts your units so in 10 seconds, you're done. I've named it "Easy Thyroid Lab Converter" and it's posted at both of my websites, *www.ScriptEssentials.com/ThyroidConverter* and *www.SuzyCohen.com/ ThyroidConverter.* In addition to this Free T3/rT3 ratio, it's good to evaluate your antibody levels to see if your thyroid is on fire.

Right now, I'm going to outline the top 5 reasons for why you've been misdiagnosed. This may look more complicated than it really is, I want to give you all the details I can because I realize you may take this into your physician. You have to become thyroid smart to become thyroid healthy!

The #1 Reason

Thyroid Hormone Is Locked Outside the Cell!

It's hard to prove this with a test because both the thyroid and pituitary glands would be behaving normally, while a trillion cells are starving for thyroid hormones. It's basically what I've been describing in most of my book and it's extremely common. It's a problem with cell receptors and they get damaged from stress which produces too much cortisol. The cells are harmed by high inflammatory cytokines like homocysteine, histamine, C Reactive protein, homocysteine, TNFα and a variety of inter-leukins. Those are all discussed in my Headache Free book.

What if your cell membranes are not healthy? The receptor sites (doorways leading inside the cell) are damaged! Bad news, then the thyroid transporters can't get across the cell membrane easily with the thyroid hormone. Your cells are starving for thyroid hormone. This is the equivalent of having a fridge full of food but the door is jammed and you can't get anything to eat. Remember, you want the thyroid hormone inside the cell, not out in your bloodstream. The membranes get damaged in people with reduced phosphatidylcholine, in people with MTHFR methylation problems, and those with deficiencies of vitamin C, or SAMe (S adenosylmethionine). For this reason, you may benefit from supplements of vitamin C, phosphatidylcholine, or SAMe. I like a specialty product that is called "ATP Fuel" by Researched Nutritionals because it contains natural ingredients that nourish your poor, weary cell membranes making everything you take work better. It's an expensive product but it might be worth it for some of you. Your doctor can order this for you, or you can look online. Adrenal adaptogenic herbs will also be helpful. Balancing hormones with something like I3C will calm down the estrogen, and that will be helpful in reducing rT3, which in turn improves your thyroid activity.

Lab results that cause this misdiagnosis: TSH and T4 are usually normal, high rT3, TBG may be low/normal, Free T3 may be normal to high (leading your doctor to say you are fine). The rT3 being elevated is not a good thing, it can be increased because of nutritional deficiencies, high cortisol (stress), high levels of antibodies made against your thyroid gland, and excessive amounts of estrogen.

The #2 Reason

You Have Been Dealing with a Lot of Stress.
You may have an undiagnosed (active) infection, blood sugar imbalances, pre-diabetes, chronic stress or have been pregnant

recently. The stress of these conditions wears out your pituitary gland so it no longer sends out the signal to the thyroid gland to make thyroxine (T4). Your pituitary gland is compromised but your thyroid gland is fine and therefore the TSH will be normal. I'm worried you will be handed a prescription for Lexapro (or some other antidepressant) when what you really need is thyroid hormone!

Lab results that cause this misdiagnosis: Normal TSH, elevated cortisol, possible high insulin or glucose abnormalities, low Free T3, elevated rT3. Not all of these will show up, but if some do, it's likely you fit in this category.

The #3 Reason

You Can't Activate Your Thyroid Hormone.

In this situation, you have poor conversion of T4 to T3 so your body isn't using what you produce. Almost all (about 90%) of the thyroid hormone your gland secretes is T4 (thyroxine) which is inactive. It's like a snack bar that is toted around in your body to where it's needed, and then eventually unwrapped and eaten (converted to T3). Becoming thyroid sick from this problem is the result of chronic stress, infection, fibromyalgia, and other problems where the cortisol is still high. In this case, your cell membranes need repair and support. Your gut also needs attention, because this problem may be due to malabsorption in the intestines, a problem that results from many things including poor probiotic status, parasite infection, H. pylori, bacterial, yeast infection, Celiac disease, or history of gastric bypass. If you have pernicious anemia that has not been detected, you will also fall into this category. Sixteen percent of Celiacs also have pernicious anemia, it's actually pretty common.

Lab results that cause the misdiagnosis: Normal TSH, T4 is normal, Free T3 is low, cytokines maybe high or normal, adrenal function could be low (or normal if malabsorption is present).

The #4 Reason

You Take "The Pill" Or Drink from Plastic Water Bottles!

You have too many transporters! They've gone and have hitched on to your thyroid hormone (making it less available to get inside the cell to revitalize you). It's caused by spikes in a protein called "thyroid binding globulin" or TBG which is one of your transporters for thyroid hormone. TBG shuttles inactive T4 around in the blood (as if it were some kind of a snack bar) thus making it unavailable to your cells. TBG and T4 are like inseparable buddies in this case. When TBG is high, Free T3 is low and you will have symptoms of hypothyroidism, more specifically you are "thyroid sick." This is commonly associated with estrogen dominance, or high estrogen from oral contraceptives (or shots/patches) and menopausal medications (Estradiol, Premarin, etc). So TBG is like a shuttle bus for thyroid hormone and it's increased from high estrogen (not good for you), and it's reduced by natural testosterone (good for you). So you want TBG to be in normal range, not high. The higher the TBG, the more T3 latches on to it, meaning lowered thyroid activity for you (because your T3 is all tied up to TBG).

The TBG can get too high if you take high doses of estrogenic herbs such as black cohosh, flax seed, kudzu, purananin, diadzein, genistein, soy milk, soy supplements, etc. The more estrogen you take in, the less likely you can break it all down properly. Hypothyroidism is a risk factor for premature birth, low birth weight, miscarriage and poor fetal neurological development so it is very important for women who are or plan to become pregnant to optimize thyroid function. Read Chapter 15, *PMS, Pregnancy and Infertility.*

Speaking of estrogen and safety, this will blow your mind but if you drink from plastic water bottles, you're estrogen levels go up from the compounds in the plastic (Bisphenol A or BPA). What if you eat commercial meat and dairy that has hormones in it, those hormones are estrogenic. Can you break it all down? I'm not so sure. Women who are too estrogenic have fibroids, heavy periods, PMS (premenstrual) problems, endometriosis and shifts in mood.

Let's assume you have poor detoxification, because you probably do. Most people do. I'm not referring to your bowel movements here, but if you're constipated, that's a problem too. When I say "poor detoxification" I mean the way your liver and kidneys clear estrogen and other chemicals, and the way your gut uses probiotics to break down food and process and eliminate toxins. There's a lot that can go wrong here. If you have any methylation problems, or other genetic snps (pronounced "snips") then these mutations will cause you to have even worse detoxification. Methylation problems are associated with attention deficit, bipolar disease, recurrent miscarriages, Down's syndrome and schizophrenia.

Methylation is responsible in part, for detoxification. If you don't methylate, you don't feel well. You can test with any lab to see if you have this genetic snp. If you do, you can be thyroid sick, even with a perfect TSH, and so you will get misdiagnosed again. You will need thyroid hormone medications, as well as something like Calcium D glucarate to package up some of these poisons and get them out of your gut. Probiotics will be a must. They convert 20% of your T4 to T3 thyroid hormone, waking you up pretty nicely. My favorite is Dr. Ohhira's Probiotic, sold nationwide.

Lab results that cause the misdiagnosis: TSH and T4 are usually normal, low Free T3, TBG is elevated, and T3 uptake is elevated.

The #5 Reason

Transporters Are All on Break!

This is the opposite of the situation above. This leaves most all of your thyroid hormone in the bloodstream for too long and your cells become resistant. There's more than an ample supply of thyroid hormone, it's just that the cells can't use it because the transporters are out to lunch! If your cells can't take it in, you still have hypothyroid symptoms. In women, this is often caused by abnormal sex hormones, such as high testosterone. You may also see PCOS (Polycystic Ovary Syndrome) blood sugar problems, high insulin or insulin resistance. Correcting the insulin and blood sugar problems will often correct the thyroid abnormalities.

Lab results that cause the misdiagnosis: TSH and T4 are often normal or even high (does that surprise you?!) The T3 is normal or elevated, TBG is slow, T3 uptake is low. (Doctors: The alpha 1 and 2 receptors that pick up the signal from T3 are also blocked by inflammatory cytokines.)

Part III
Drug Muggers

Chapter 7

Restore Mugged Nutrients

Step 3 of my "Script" to get you well is to restore mugged nutrients. In order to become thyroid healthy, you need to have all the nutrients available to make thyroid hormone, then activate it. Drugs steal nutrients from your body, either by using them up during absorption or by directly interfering with their activation. Statin cholesterol drugs take out CoQ10 causing the infamous liver problems and muscle cramps. Birth control pills deplete probiotics and magnesium leading to vaginal yeast infections and depression. Those pills can take out zinc too, leading to hypothyroidism. Acid blocking pills and antacids are drug muggers for so many nutrients that they can lead to 100s of new diseases but those "diseases" are really just nutrient depletions. This drug mugging effect can explain everything from nagging aches to life-threatening diseases, and for our purposes here, it means that certain drugs you take (or foods or beverages you consume) are "mugging" nutrients from your body.

Being deficient in key nutrients will never be fixed by medicine. I'm so passionate about nutrient deficiencies and how our body becomes depleted by taking medications that I wrote the book on it! It's called Drug Muggers (Rodale 2011) and it's available in various languages. Little did I know this book (originally self-published) and written by myself on the floor of my living room with my 'desk' (a cardboard box from Storage Containers) would go on to become an international best-seller and number one in it's category! This book solves so many problems for people who are really healthier than they think. It's your side effect solution.

What you may not realize is that one drug causes side effects, and you get diagnosed with a disease because of that side effect, and then medicated with one drug after another. This problem is solved if you know what the side effects are from the first drug, and I tell you those secrets! I help you to restore lost nutrients in Drug Muggers so that you don't accidentally get medicated for 3 diseases you don't really have. For our purposes here, I want you to know that if you don't have some essential vitamins, minerals and cofactors in your body you can't make thyroid hormone causing hypothyroidism. Let's say you DO have what you need on board to make thyroxine (T4) but you don't have what you need to transport it into the cell. That makes you thyroid sick.

To give you an example, zinc is classically mugged by oral contraceptives, and so long term use of these pills causes a deficiency of zinc. If you have low zinc you can't convert T4 to T3, and that means low thyroid hormone, which can cause hair loss or thinning. Another example of drug mugging is with acid reducing medications (and also coffee), which reduces magnesium. You need magnesium along with thyroid hormone to make your heart beat, and create ATP, our body's fuel. A deficiency of magnesium leads to muscle pain, fatigue and heartbeat rhythm disturbances. Here are the ways you can become nutrient deficient and thus, hypothyroid (or thyroid sick):

1. Not eating nutrient dense foods
2. Deficient in digestive enzymes
3. Poor probiotic status which you need to extract nutrients
4. Gastrointestinal infections
5. Low gastric acidity
6. Poor iron, magnesium and iodine
7. Celiac disease
8. Irritable bowel syndrome

9. Chronic diarrhea
10. Taking birth control
11. Glutamine deficiency

If you eat a nutritionally naked diet of refined foods, you deplete your minerals then you can't convert that T4 to precious T3, which is what so many of you need to do. This becomes particularly important for people who take the drug Levothyroxine (Synthroid) because that drug is pure T4. You must (*repeat, you must*) convert that T4 to T3 inside the cell, or you will remain in sleepy, hibernation mode! And you need the nutrients to do that. If you're taking some popular drugs that deplete nutrients, you cannot effectively convert to T3, until you put back what medication stole. It's not just drugs, there are other thyroid thieves, refer to Chapter 8, *Thyroid Thieves Lurking Everywhere.*

Thyroid Healthy Tip

No matter how much thyroid medicine you take, it will NEVER get activated or into your cells unless you have adequate levels of minerals. Surprise, coffee is a drug mugger of minerals so you are likely deficient if you drink it! You don't have to give up coffee, I'm not a meanie. I'm just saying to replenish your mineral stash by eating mineral-rich greens, or taking trace mineral supplements. Separate administration from your thyroid medicine by 4 hours. Got it? Good, because your happiness and waistline are at stake.

Nutritional Deficiencies that Block T4 to T3 Conversion

Be mindful of your diet and be sure to include the following nutrients which are all needed to convert T4 to T3. If you're missing even one of these from a poor diet then you're apt to have sluggish thyroid conversion. To get you thyroid healthy, we have to have these guys on board!

+ Vitamin A
+ Chromium
+ Vitamin D
+ Iodine
+ Iron
+ Vitamin B12 (methylcobalamin)
+ Pyridoxal 5' Phosphate (the active form of vitamin B6)
+ Vitamin B2 (riboflavin)
+ Selenium
+ Zinc

When you take a drug mugger of a nutrient needed to convert that drug, you don't get the full benefits of the drug. Now, I'm going to share an important detail, one rarely spoken: If you have high levels of rT3 do not take T4 drugs because you'll tend to make more rT3, thus making yourself worse. Remember that!

Table 8. Drug Mugging Effect On Your Thyroid

There is a more comprehensive explanation of each thyroid and a list of dozens of drugs that mug each of these nutrients in my other book, Drug Muggers.

Symptom	Nutrient Deficiency
Cravings	Chromium
Hair loss	Zinc
Dry Skin	Vitamin A
Fatigue	Iron and riboflavin
Weight	Probiotics
Depression	Vitamin D
Infections	Selenium
Insomnia	Melatonin
Pain	Magnesium

You can order a lab test which requires blood. This is often referred to "micronutrient" testing. For pennies a day, you can find out what micronutrients are low. These labs are just guidelines, and while I'm recommending them, I wouldn't put my life in the hands of a blood test. It's really about the clinical picture for me. So if you take a test that says your low in B12 (methylcobalamin) or zinc as another example, I'd look up the symptoms associated with those deficiencies just to see if I had them. If I didn't, I wouldn't supplement. We are so unique, and we have to customize our regimen to what works best for us.

For example, if you take fluoxetine (Prozac) or statin cholesterol drugs, you may be deficient in iodine, which means you can't make T4 (thyroxine). The reason is because fluoride (in those drugs) is a drug mugger of iodine. If you take oral contraceptives and you're short on zinc as a result of the drug mugging effect, you can't convert T4 to T3 well, see what I mean? It's a problem. For a complete list of all the drug nutrient depletions and how to correct them, please refer to my Drug Muggers book sold on Amazon. If you're taking a drug mugger and you don't replenish with what you're losing each day, then expect these so-called side effects of these deficiencies go on to get diagnosed as a new disease! You'll get on a medication merry-go-round and it's a hard ride to get off.

In the meantime, I've outlined several nutrients here so that you can get started with the absolute crucial ones. Up first is selenium because that is fundamental to getting you "thyroid healthy."

Selenium Deficiencies Lead to Thyroid Illness

Selenium is a mineral with strong antioxidant powers, and it is one of the most important minerals for your thyroid gland. Autoimmune thyroid disorders worsen in the presence of low selenium. One study in the *Journal of Rheumatology* showed a 40% reduction in antibodies against the thyroid, by improving selenium.

People with digestive or bowel problems like Celiac disease, Crohn's and IBS (irritable bowel syndrome) will run out of this mineral quickly. Deficiencies can lead to thyroid problems of all sorts, heart disease, exhaustion, and poor immune function.

Dosage: 100–400 mcg per day; no more than 400 mcg from all your sources. I would start at 100mcg and go up from there if you need to.

Drug Muggers of Selenium
+ Corticosteroids (prednisone, dexamethasone)
+ Oral contraceptives
+ Hormone replacement therapy (Estrace, Climara, conjugated estrogens like Premarin)
+ Asthma and Allergy inhalers (like Flonase, Advair, etc)
+ Many antibiotics
+ Diabetic medications

Iron Deficiencies Lead to Thyroid Illness

Iron deficiency leads to very poor T4 to T3 conversion, so you become clinically hypothyroid which slows metabolism. The net result is weight gain. You may think you're tired because you have low iron, and less oxygen is carried around your body, but you're probably not terribly anemic, it's more likely that you are "thyroid sick" due to the poor T3 activity. The reason I'm bringing this up is because the *World Health Organization* (WHO) estimates that 2 billion people (30%) of the world's population now are anemic as a result of iron deficiency. That's a lot of people walking around with thyroid disease that probably don't know it. You may be anemic if you are vegan or vegetarian, if you have low stomach acid, heavy periods, kidney disease, or have a minor perforation in the GI tract. Take a look at all the drugs that mug iron from your body. Top of the list is coffee and tea (not herbal tea).

Dosage: 20–30mg elemental per day; Iron bisglycinate is among the best because it is easy on the stomach, however like all iron pills, it should be taken with food. No more than 30mg from all your sources.

Drug Muggers of Iron

+ Coffee and tea
+ Acid blockers (esomeprazole, omeprazole, famotidine, ranitidine, etc)
+ Antacids (Maalox, Mylanta)
+ Antibiotics
+ Blood pressure meds of ACE Inhibitor class (captopril, enalapril, lisinopril)
+ Oral contraceptives
+ Hormone replacement therapy (Estrace, Climara, conjugated estrogens like Premarin)
+ Cholestyramine resin
+ Furosemide
+ HCTZ or hydrochlorothiazide (any drug containing this)
+ Levonorgestrel (in birth control)
+ Norethindrone (found in many birth control pills)
+ SERMs for breast cancer (raloxifene, tamoxifen and others)
+ Excessive calcium supplementation

Cautions for Iron- You must determine the dosage with your physician. It can cause harmless discoloration of your stool, and it's highly constipating. One of the best forms is iron bisglycinate because it's easier on the tummy. Some people can drink orange juice each day and that increases absorption of iron from your foods so you don't have to take a supplement; that's nice because iron is hard on the stomach and causes constipation. In most cases, this is not enough. A typical dose would be 20 to 30 mg per day until your ferritin rises. You do not take this at the same time as your thyroid, separate administration by 4 to 6 hours. Don't take iron supplements with dairy. Low iron may be tied to H. pylori gut infections, talk to your gastroenterologist about this. Finally, some of you have very stubbornly low ferritin levels that do not rise for many years. I hear ya! That was me for a long time too, and the only thing that really turned that around for good was a product called ATP Fuel by Researched Nutritionals. It helps with cell membrane repair. Other things that helped me were Hawaiian Spirulina by Nutrex Hawaii and eating liver and onions! A crucial component that finally lifted the anemic veil for me was taking betaine with pepsin supplements with every meal. I was apparently hypochlorhydric and therefore, not absorbing iron from my meals. This is covered some more in Chapter 5, *The Best Lab Tests.*

Vitamin D Deficiencies Lead to Thyroid Illness

Most people know about the sunshine vitamin and how it helps keep muscles and bones strong as well as infections at bay. It's great for people who feel melancholy, especially SAD (seasonal affective disorder) and those with heart rhythm disturbances. As it pertains to the thyroid, vitamin D deficiency leads to very poor T4 to T3 conversion inside the cell, as well as higher antibodies against your thyroid gland. You're more likely to run out of D if you're a vegetarian, if you take a drug mugger, have liver or kidney disease or genetic snps.

Drug Muggers of Vitamin D

+ Acid blockers (famotidine, omeprazole, ranitidine, etc)
+ Antacids (Maalox, Mylanta)
+ Anticonvulsants (Carbamazepine, valproic acid and others)
+ Cholesterol drugs (cholestyramine, colestipol and fibrates)

✦ Statin cholesterol drugs (atorvastatin, lovastatin, etc)
✦ Ketoconazole
✦ Butalbital-containing drugs (Fiorinal, Fioricet)
✦ Calcium channel blockers (verapamilm amlodipine, nifedipine)
✦ Fluticasone (Flonase)
✦ Gabapentin (Neurontin)
✦ Laxatives that contain magnesium like "magnesium citrate" or milk of magnesia
✦ Mineral Oil
✦ Olestra (fat substitute often used in "light" potato chips)
✦ Orlistat (Alli, Xenical)
✦ OTC diet aids & Fat blockers (kidney bean extract or starch neutralizers)
✦ SERMs for breast cancer (raloxifene, tamoxifen and others)
✦ Steroids (dexamethasone, hydrocortisone, prednisone)
✦ Stimulant Laxatives

Dosage of Vitamin D: This is something you must determine with your physician. A typical dose is 2,000–10,000 IU per day until levels normalize and you can determine serum vitamin D levels with a blood test. You can take this at the same time as your thyroid in the morning if you really want to, there's no interaction. If not, just take it with breakfast or lunch. Meals improve absorption, however you should not be eating with your thyroid medicine.

Zinc Deficiencies Lead to Thyroid Illness

Some clues you have zinc deficiency include all the symptoms of thyroid illness, including hair loss or thinning, loss of taste/smell, erectile dysfunction or chronic diarrhea. Zinc is needed for your TSH hormone to work, and to help you produce T3, as opposed to rT3. Zinc helps activate thyroid hormone too. Did you know you lose zinc when you have your monthly cycle? Yes, it's lost through menstrual blood. Zinc is a strong anti-inflammatory modulator, and it helps with autoimmune thyroid illness, as well as diabetes and both those conditions go hand-in-hand many times. Here are some common medication categories that zap your zinc while you sleep, and there's a much longer list in my other book, Drug Muggers.

Drug Muggers of Zinc

+ Anti-inflammatories
+ Antibiotics
+ Acid blockers (famotidine, omeprazole, ranitidine, etc)
+ Antacids (Maalox, Mylanta)
+ Antivirals (AZT, zidovudine, lamivudine, etc)
+ Blood pressure drugs, most of them
+ Cholesterol medicines (clofibrate, fenofibrate, gemfibrozil)
+ Clonidine
+ Diuretics used for edema and blood pressure control
+ Ezetimibe
+ Furosemide
+ Oral contraceptives
+ Hormone replacement therapy (Estrace, Climara, conjugated estrogens like Premarin)
+ Methyldopa
+ SERMs for breast cancer (raloxifene, tamoxifen and others)
+ The condition of "estrogen dominance"
+ Casein, the protein in dairy
+ Chocolate, it's high in copper which reduces zinc if you eat too much
+ Smoking

Dosage of Zinc: This is something you must determine with your physician. A typical dose is 15–50 mg per day until levels normalize. You do not take this at the same time as your thyroid, separate administration by 4 to 6 hours.

Have Enough Bs on Board?

Do you have pins and needles nerve pain, depression, fatigue, anemia or weight gain? This could be related to a deficiency of B vitamins. Your stash gets depleted by female hormones (menopause and birth control), antacids, ulcer medications, diuretics used for blood pressure, raloxifene, cholestyramine, diabetic drugs and tea and coffee.

Put Back What Medication Stole

As you can see, there are hundreds of medications that rob your body, and even foods and beverages do it too. It's rare when a drug mugger causes classical "hypothyroidism," more often the deficiencies cause you to be "thyroid sick" because you can't use your T4, nor can you activate it. If you are taking multiple medications on this list, including thyroid medications, then you need to replenish all the deficient nutrients. The best way to do that is with a combination of the following:

1. Probiotics
2. Trace minerals
3. B complex

The order in which this is done is as follows. You would take your probiotics in the morning with your thyroid medication and a full glass of water. If you are taking your probiotics twice daily then take the second dose at bedtime. When taking trace minerals, take those with any meal of the day to reduce stomach upset and enhance absorption. The B complex can be taken any time during the day too, preferably with a meal. Because those sometimes spark some energy, it's ideal to take them anytime before 4 or 5 o'clock at night. If taking three different supplements feels overwhelming, or the timing is difficult for you, another plan is to take a medical grade foods which combine a lot of different nutrients plus protein (like rice, pea, hemp or whey). This should be taken anytime, so long as it is 2 hours or more after you take your thyroid medication. There is much more about the dosing and instructions in my Drug Muggers book, available on Amazon.

Chapter 8

Thyroid Thieves Lurking Everywhere

In chemistry there is a group of elements called halogens. Of all the halogens, the most dangerous is fluorine, followed by chlorine, then bromine, then iodine. There's one more called astatine, but it's rare. Of the halogens, iodine is the good guy because it makes thyroid hormone. The fluorine, chlorine and bromine are the bad halogens and if you look on a periodic table, you'll see they are lined up as relatives of each other in the same group. When they are biochemically reduced, their name changes slightly and they become "halides" such as iodide, bromide, fluoride, and chloride.

Your thyroid gland concentrates iodine, the others are considered toxic to the gland. The thyroid has a powerful pump that concentrates it 50 to 100 fold over the blood. Halogens, like fluoride will be taken up like a sponge. Your thyroid gland sees fluoride, but because it looks like beloved iodine, it gets sucked in. Bad news now, you can't make thyroid hormone. Think of yourself answering the doorbell and letting the thief inside your home because that thief looked just like your loved one!

What makes the bad guys (fluorine, chlorine and bromine) so very bad is that they are bullies. They bully iodine and chase it out of your thyroid gland. The bromine, fluorine and chlorine are all known to compete and take the place of iodine wherever iodine needs to go. Just FYI, iodine needs to go to your reproductive organs (breasts, uterus, testicles, prostate). For our purposes, iodine needs to be available to make thyroid hormone, so if it's displaced with bromine bullies (or chlorine or fluorine) then you can't make enough T4, or T3. Hello hypothyroidism!

Fluorine or Fluoride

This is a common thyroid thief and it's often found in tap water, but it depends where you live. You can remove much of the fluoride by putting a filter on your tap. Unfortunately, fluoride is in toothpaste, mouthwash and other dental products. It is known to assault your pineal gland (which, when left undisturbed by fluoride, makes sufficient amounts of sleep hormone melatonin). Fluoride is slippery, and easily absorbed through skin and mucus membranes, so it can definitely get up into your pineal gland. It can get into your thyroid too, and displace iodine. How are you supposed to make T4 out of tyrosine (that's the "T" part) and 4 atoms of fluoride? You absolutely cannot do it! You need 4 atoms of iodine, not fluoride! Do you see how using fluoride-free personal care products might help you make more thyroid hormone? It's because fluoride can displace iodine from your thyroid cells, and then you can't make thyroid hormone. I told you some of these halogens were bullies!

Fluoride has huge medical use, and I'm not being sarcastic. It was the treatment of choice to shut down the gland when overactive! Yes, it was, and it still works that way! It's medical use is to suppress thyroid activity, and can be used as an effective strategy to help people with hyperthyroidism (like Graves'). It's excellent treatment for Graves' disease. Putting a thyroid suppressing drug like fluoride in tap water doesn't make sense to me. It's really unfair, it could make you hypothyroid.

Fluoride is in a lot of dental products including toothpaste, but there's not enough to cause damage with one toothbrushing. Over the years, if you swallow enough, it's going to be a problem because we can't get around the issue that fluoride is a known poison to the thyroid gland. It even says to call 9-1-1- if you swallow toothpaste right there on the label. So I do suggest you avoid fluoride toothpaste, there are plenty of fluoride-free alternatives. But toothpaste is really nothing compared to fluorinated drugs like the quinolones! These go by brand names Cipro, Levaquin and Avelox, among others. I just want you to be extra extra cautious and avoid anything that harms your precious thyroid so I usually suggest cephalosporins or macrolide antibiotics instead of the quinolones. For more information regarding quinolone antibiotics refer to Table 9 Could Your Fluorinated Drug Crash Your Thyroid? Keep in mind some of these drugs are still on the market, but there were many others and they were withdrawn by the Food and Drug Administration.

Table 9. Could Your Fluorinated Drug Crash Your Thyroid?
These medications have a fluoride backbone from which they are derived: Atorvastatin (Lipitor) Citalopram (Celexa) Dexamethasone (Decadron) Escitalopram (Lexapro) Fluconazole (Diflucan) Flunisolide (Nasarel, Nasalide, AeroBid) Fluororoquinolone antibiotics (Cipro, Levaquin, Avelox) Fluoxetine (Prozac) Flurazepam (Dalmane) Fluticasone (Flonase) Fluvastatin (Lescol) Fluvoxamine (Luvox) Lansoprazole (Prevacid) Midazolam (Versed) Omeprazole (Prilosec) Paroxetine (Paxil)

Bromine or Bromide

Bromine (sometimes referred to as bromide) is present in a number of foods including bread and other baked goods and sodas. It's seen as brominated vegetable oil or BVO and has been used since the 1930s to help suspend the flavors in the water. It's used as an emulsifier to stabilize sodas like Mountain Dew and some energy drinks. In an article by Dr. Joseph Mercola, this soda and all its ingredients, was referred to as "A weapon of mass destruction, in a can."

It was used in Gatorade until January 2013, when Pepsico finally took it out but they still keep it in the Mountain Dew (as of this writing). Baked goods and some flours may contain potassium bromate which is a dough conditioner. Check labels for bromide or brominated compounds and avoid!

Medications contain a form of bromine too. Some are Atrovent Inhaler, Atrovent Nasal Spray, Pro-Banthine (for ulcers), and anesthesia agents. Bromine poisoning can cause paranoid schizophrenia and all sorts of psychiatric problems. If you are ingesting too much, it could cause severe acne, skin rash, fatigue, abdominal pain, cardiac arrhythmias and a metallic taste in your mouth.

Halogen Light Bulbs

I can't find a study that says these harm your thyroid gland. I really am all about the environment, however these light bulbs worry me if you have thyroid illness.

You see, halogen light bulbs utilize a closed capsule (fused quartz envelope) allowing for higher temperatures. That's their claim to fame. But inside the quartz envelope is a vapor of argon and a halogen. It was originally iodine, but now it's usually bromine. Replacing these bulbs may not be a bad idea but keep in mind, bromine is more commonly found in your food supply, than in your bulbs.

Chlorine or Chloride

Tap Water? Oh No! It contains fluoride most of the time which reduces thyroid levels, and it also contains chlorine as a disinfected. This makes a tap water filter particularly important because you don't want to consume too much chlorine. It goes through your skin so if you are a swimmer or love hot tubs (laden with chlorine), you may need extra iodine in your diet or supplement. I could go on and on about chlorine, it's in bleach, it's in your shower (get a filter), it's in cleansers.

Organochlorine compounds are controversial and many experts think they lower thyroid hormone or damage the gland (Environmental Health Perspectives 1999) The term "organochlorine compound" means the compound has an organic compound with a covalent carbon-chlorine bond. Pharmaceuticals sometimes contain this chlorine or are synthesized with a chlorine compound. Chlorine is essential to the manufacture of about 93% of the world's best-selling drugs. What do they do to your thyroid gland? I'm not 100% sure because some drugs are manufactured with the help of chlorine so they don't contain chlorine at all. Other drugs are chlorine-based, so they contain a molecule, or several molecules which I have noted for you with an asterisk:

* Amlodipine (Norvasc) for blood pressure
Acid blockers (Prevacid, Nexium, Pepcid, Zantac)
Advair diskus for asthma
* Chlordiazepoxide (Librium) a sedative
* Chloral hydrate, a strong sedative/hypnotic
* Chlorpheniramine (Chlor-Trimeton) the antihistamine
* Clopidogrel (Plavix) used for blood thinning
* Glucovance for diabetes
Lamotrigine (Lamictal) the anticonvulsant
Loratadine (Claritin) the antihistamine
Olanzapine (Zyprexa) a psychotropic drug

* Splenda the artificial sweetener
* Sertraline (Zoloft) the antidepressant
Statin cholesterol reducing medications (Lipitor, Zocor)
* Venlafaxine
* Vancomycin, an antibiotic

Put Down the Plastic

Many people drink from water bottles while jogging or
when eating out. It's almost a way of life for some
people. It contains a problematic compound. Bisphenol
A blocks the thyroid receptors (doorways) into your cell
all over your body (but not in the pituitary). The net
result is that your labs look okay to your doctor (because
the TSH is normal) but you are really thyroid resistant,
or thyroid sick as I've been referring to it.

Sodium chloride has ionic sodium-chloride bonds and is a
chloride salt—a very different material from an organochlorine.
Sodium chloride will dissolve in water, breaking the ionic bond,
to give sodium ions and chloride ions; both are common in the
environment and relatively harmless. Carbon-chlorine covalent
bonds will not break when the compound is dissolved, whether
in fat (nonpolar) or water (polar).

But, organochlorine is a very broad category of compounds
and it would be far too generalized to say that all organochlorine
compounds have similar behavior in the human body. Certainly,
the structures being discussed here are quite varied. From a
cursory glance, I'd say that the major thing that the organochlorine compounds mentioned here have in common is that they are
relatively nonpolar, which would make them soluble in fats
(although some, like Splenda, are also water soluble).

Avoid the Poison

You must make a concerted effort to eliminate fluorine, chlorine and bromine from your diet, your environment and your body in order for iodine to be fully available to your thyroid cells. For me, I avoid these chemicals as much as possible but sometimes it's hard, like if I want to go swimming during the summertime. There is chlorine in the pool, and lots of it. When you take a shower in a hotel (or even your own home) there is chlorine in the water, unless you have a filter to remove it. When I feel like I've had a heavy exposure of a halogen, I take one capsule of i-Throid or one tablet of Iodoral, whatever I have in my house. I don't stay on it forever, I just take one that day, and maybe one more a week later because in my mind, that restores some of my lost iodine. I think we are all a little iodine deficient, but I would test first to be 100% sure.

The point is, if you do not make a concerted effort, your iodine gets wasted by these bullies and your thyroxine production goes down. Iodine deficiency affects your reproductive organs. If you didn't know what I just taught you in this chapter, your practitioner may keep pumping you full of medicine. There's a more intelligent way to handle thyroid illness than to keep taking the next best drug (and higher doses of each one). It's much more effective if you clear your body of toxins, contaminants, thyroid-suppressing halogens, and other inflammation-causing foods and poisons. That is a wonderful way to protect your body. The only exception to this rule of thumb is for people who have had their thyroid gland surgically removed. You will need life-long thyroid hormone replenishment.

Chapter 9

Mistakes Prevent You from Getting Thyroid Healthy

My book is about empowerment. I'm determined to educate you so well about your thyroid condition that you can speak in such a way that 'gets the job done,' by that I mean, gets you feeling thyroid healthy. Enough is enough, you know?! So this next section is devoted to teaching you about mistakes and assumptions made, that prevent you from getting thyroid healthy. If you know the mistakes made in clinics around the country, then you will be better able to address them head on if they happen to you. Here are the 10 most common errors made at the doctor's office, and one of the reasons you still feel awful even though you take medication for years:

1. They measure thyroxine (T4 levels) in the serum. This does not speak to the levels inside your cells (tissues). What's in the blood is NOT in the cell (because it's in the blood!)

2. Physicians try to verify your thyroid status with TSH blood tests and when those come back normal, they dismiss you. Bad news! You have to fight for your life then. Some people with thyroid disease do better on medication, regardless of their tests. Convincing your

physician to treat you anyway could make the difference. Many disorders are treated on the "clinical presentation" because the tests are not validated, for example fibromyalgia, CFIDS (chronic fatigue immunodeficiency syndrome), Lyme disease and others.

3. Having thyroid disease is limited to the thyroid gland. This is woefully incorrect. Thyroid hormone supports every single cell in your body and all your organs. You have to optimize thyroid function or you'll feel terrible head to toe. Low levels of thyroid hormone, specifically T3, comes with a higher risk of mortality so you're going to die sooner than someone who has optimal levels. This is a life-giving hormone that works head to toe. The lower your T3, the higher your risk of death.

4. They didn't measure your Reverse T3 (rT3). It's assumed that rT3 is meaningless since it does not have biological activity like T3 but nothing could be further from the truth. The importance of rT3 cannot be underestimated. When it's high, it prevents the cell from taking up the active thyroid hormone. Your cells starve for T3 because neither Free T3 or rT3 can get in, because the rT3 is hooked on! If you're cells could speak, they'd say to the rT3 "Get off already, my body is freezing cold and I'm tired, depressed and heavy! For God sakes, GET OFF!" Evaluating rT3 will give you an indication of cellular hunger. If the level of rT3 is high, you need thyroid medicine, and not a T4 drug (that won't work), you'll need either T3, or a combination of T4 and T3 like Natural Desiccated Thyroid.

5. Your TPO was normal. It's assumed that if you have normal antibodies for TPO (thyroperoxidase), that your thyroid is not inflamed or being attacked. Big mistake because that is just one popular marker. There are other

antibodies that can be evaluated and tested with your blood. You may have some other antibody that is high, causing inflammation and destruction of your gland so you need to test for others.

6. No one is addressing your impaired gut function. It's assumed that when you take a medication you will absorb it but if you have impaired gut function, an undiagnosed infection or low acid in your stomach, then you will not get the full benefit of your medication. Heal the gut first, and your medication will work much better. So will your supplements.

7. You're inactivating your medicine with supplements. There are interactions between thyroid supplements and thyroid medicines. Sometimes, supplements contain minerals that tie up your thyroid medicine and take it out. Separate administration of supplements by 2 to 4 hours unless it's a probiotic, then you can take it at the same time. Interactions don't always mean lowered activity of thyroid medicine, it can be the opposite. You can take supplements that jack up your thyroid dose, and that is real dangerous. For example, there are some herbal supplements that contain actual thyroid hormone (like in a tainted supplement, or in a glandular supplement), and this spikes drug levels which could lead to a thyroid storm. You have to be extremely choosy about what supplements you buy, and what they contain. Don't make the mistake of assuming that just because a supplement is sold without a prescription that it's safe, or that it's right for you.

8. You're drinking soy milk. Don't assume that soy is good for you. It's all the health rage, especially with vegetarians and vegans, but soy protein powders, soy isoflavones and menopause supplement that contain

high amounts of soy (or soy derived genistein for
example) can crash your thyroid levels. That is why
they are termed "goitrogens" because they can cause a
goiter, which is the swelling of the neck because of an
enlarged thyroid gland. The gland swells sometimes
because of low iodine too. I don't recommend soybean
oil either, it's not good for your thyroid. Soy is often
genetically modified too, you won't find anything in
my kitchen with it.

9. You're taking a weight-loss aid or fitness supplement
   containing L-carnitine. This is a supplement that I
   love but high amounts of it can reduce the activity of
   thyroid hormone and calm things down, that's why it's
   used in Graves' disease. Please don't be afraid of it, it's
   excellent, just don't take a lot. L-carnitine is an amino
   acid important for cardiac health and body-building.
   The acetylated version, as in Acetyl L carnitine, which
   I recommend for brain fog and memory problems
   because it creates some acetylcholine in the brain (a
   memory molecule).

10. You're taking minerals at the same time as your thyroid
    medication. Minerals especially calcium, iron, iodine
    or magnesium, or a multi-mineral supplement, needs
    to be spaced away by 4 to 6 hours from your thyroid
    medicine. Preferably, take the thyroid hormone upon
    arising in the morning on an empty stomach, and take
    the mineral supplements with food at lunch or dinner.
    Many of you take iodine supplements. Just so you
    know, these don't make your thyroid hormone work
    better in the cell, but they do help create more thyroxine
    (T4). If you need iodine, it's okay to take those without
    regard to medication time.

Part IV
Thyroid Associated Illness

Chapter 10

Weight Gain

Don't blame yourself for holding on to weight, or for gaining it. We are addicted to the chemicals in food, this has been known for decades. The food industry puts more sugar in seemingly healthy foods than in some of our junk foods! All the while you are resisting temptations like gooey doughnuts, greasy cheeseburgers and soda you're getting it in certain brands of natural juice, milk, applesauce and vitamin infused water. You have to become neurotic like me and read every label of every food product you want to eat. If you don't, you will put on unsuspecting weight, then have to diet, and this cycle becomes a yo-yo. If you feel heavy and tired, it's probably due to low thyroid and high leptin. You can measure leptin with a blood test.

What Is Leptin?

Leptin is a hormone that has a strong bearing on how much thyroid hormone is produced by your thyroid gland. Leptin is technically a protein that's made in fat cells, and it's good for you. Leptin is your 'stop sign' for eating. When your body secretes leptin, you start to feel full, not that you stop eating (because there's always room for dessert right?) but leptin gives you that sense of satiety and you should listen to it. When you get that sense of fullness caused by leptin, step away from the fork!

Pay attention to leptin! If you don't, you become leptin resistant. Then, no matter how much leptin is secreted from your cells, your brain doesn't see the signal to stop eating, it thinks there's a famine going on. Just like Pavlov's dog, you become conditioned. In this case, you see the hormone leptin but ignore it, and keep eating. It causes resistance.

What Is Leptin & Leptin Resistance?

With leptin resistance, your brain thinks your body is starving. I know this sounds ridiculous to you, but it is very common, dare I say epidemic, and it affects your thyroid gland badly! When you're thyroid gland gets involved, your risk for headaches goes up. Refer to my *Headache Free* book, for more on that.

When leptin resistance happens in the body, it basically 'tells' your thyroid gland via complex signaling hormones to slow down metabolism and stop burning food for calories. In other words, it tells you to hold on to fat to survive the famine (remember it thinks you are starving to death).

Leptin Resistance = Fat Storage

Whenever you go on a diet, and then come off of it, leptin commands that any calories from the food you now eat (after the diet) get stored as fat in case starvation sets in again (it's really afraid you're going to go on another crash diet). You see, your body doesn't know that your diet is over with for good, it thinks at any time you are going to start dramatically cutting calories again, so it wants to make sure you don't die. Even if you eat like a bird, you still hold on to weight. Your brain and thyroid are 'terrified' that at any given moment, you will go back into starvation mode again (the next new diet), so the hormone sends signals to start padding your hips and belly with some fat just in case food becomes scarce. This is why yo-yo dieting is bad.

Leptin and Lab Results

To confuse matters, and doctors who evaluate your thyroid status is that T3 falls while you're starving yourself on someone's new crazy diet. At the same time, Reverse T3 (rT3) increases, blocking your natural thyroid hormone's effect and further slowing your metabolism. Simply put, your thyroid hormones go so far out of whack that you put on weight but the standard conventional blood tests (TSH and T4) don't pick that up, you'll be told you're "normal" and sent home with all your hypothyroidism symptoms, and no plan to help you lose weight or feel better. So so sad, it makes me mad in fact. That's why I'm trying so hard to help you here. I want you to really get this, so you can have a conversation with those in charge of your health and get proper treatment. The TSH test is completely unreliable in overweight people with a leptin that is elevated. Don't even spend your money on it. Save your money to buy some medication to kick start your metabolism again. Leptin resistance inflames the thyroid gland. Do you recall how bad inflammatory cytokines are? They are one primary cause of thyroid disease (and other diseases). I firmly believe pro-inflammatory cytokines are a major cause for illness, pain and cancer. Hashi sufferers frequently have some degree of leptin resistance.

Edit What You Eat

I don't recommend crash dieting. Slow and steady is the name of the game. Why do you think we have hundreds of diet books, as a general rule? Rarely do they work. I always say to "edit" what you eat, don't "diet." It's a play on the letters of those two words, so instead of eating apple pie, you edit what you eat, and go for the apple. Instead of potato chips, go for the potato. It's these slight edits that help you lose weight over time. Correct hormonal imbalances, and adrenal fatigue. Read the chapter "Lose Fat While You Sleep" in my first book *The 24-Hour Pharmacist* (Collins 2009) for information on how to edit what you eat and make the weight loss stick.

Walking Into Walls Lately?

Here's an interesting little-known fact! If you have poor coordination and bump into things more often than you should, this could be due to a thyroid problem, driven by leptin imbalances. When people lose weight, antibodies against the thyroid gland may return to normal. This is a good thing. You know what else reduces antibodies against the thyroid gland? Eating a gluten free diet, or preferably a completely grain free diet, like the Phase One diet, or the Paleo diet. This means no rice, quinoa, wheat, rye, spelt, amaranth, corn ... none of it! There is more information about leptin in Chapter 5, *The Best Lab Tests*. You can test for food sensitivities at CyrexLabs.com, they are the most comprehensive lab for this.

Low Thyroid Causes Diabetes

Hypothyroidism leads to insulin resistance, diabetes and metabolic syndrome, so if you have diabetes, you have to take a step back and examine thyroid tests. If you're thyroid tests are abnormal, diabetes is next. When you have diabetes, you focus on blood sugar and insulin and I'm saying that's a mistake, you have to go to the root cause, which is often undiagnosed thyroid illness. Diabetics have been shown to have 50% less conversion of T4 to T3, but usually the T4 is the only marker evaluated. Only the best physicians know to evaluate Free T3. Most physicians measure what they were taught to in school, the T4 and the TSH levels and this could cause you to fall through the cracks. You'll put on more weight, because your thyroid gland is on fire, and then one day, all of a sudden they tell you that you have diabetes. Trust me it didn't happen overnight. It was years in the making. If you have diabetes, you do not need more T4 so I'd recommend you explore other medications. T4 drugs are an inappropriate and ineffective method of treatment for insulin resistance, leptin resistance and diabetes.

I want to help you because diabetes is dangerous. The complications include heart attack, amputation, kidney failure and blindness. You might be able to prevent the diabetes if you address the thyroid condition soon enough, so testing is critical. Just FYI, the very medications and insulin shots used for diabetes can cause more weight gain and they do not enhance or heal your thyroid! I've written an entire book on the subject, refer to *Diabetes without Drugs* (Rodale 2010). You will also learn much more about losing weight and protecting your heart, eyesight and limbs! This is a best-selling book, sold all around the world. It's even used in some physician's classrooms to teach them how to treat diabetes using my perspective. This is a distinction that sets my book apart from all other books on the topic.

Want to know why I'm so adamant about this? It's because the classic response given to you if you're overweight is to tell you to diet some more (which I'm telling you won't help), and to take statin cholesterol drugs! "Oy vey" like my mom would say! Dieting doesn't work with leptin resistance, but eliminating grains could, and avoiding refined sugars and bad fats. You know how to do this, and there are books on the subject. Eat like a caveman, that's basically what I'm saying. There was no soda in paleolithic times, and no boxed foods. You know how to do this, and if you're not sure, you can refer to some recipes I wrote in my *Diabetes without Drugs* book, which really helps people drop weight fast.

Leptin Levels

A leptin above 12 is considered high and I would say that you need thyroid hormone in this case, as in medications. Taking antioxidants and anti-inflammatories can help. You're more likely to have leptin resistance if you have do yo-yo diets. Some of the new medications like Byetta and Victoza may help with leptin resistance. I'm not a big fan of them, but maybe for short term.

Leptin resistance causes you to have a 25% reduced metabolism. In other words, you won't be able to turn all your food into fuel, you'll store it as fat. If you compare two people who are the same age, the same size body frame, the same body fat, then the yo yo dieters burn 25% fewer calories burned per day.

Exercise But Don't Overdo It!

Studies show too much exercise lowers metabolism especially in women. If your body senses too much "stress" and metabolism drops, then you're fighting yourself. The studies specifically show that intense exercise especially when combined with dieting slows down the production of active thyroid hormone.

There's a connection between thyroid hormone and metabolism, which translates to how skinny you are. Do you eat like a bird and still hold on to weight or gain more? It's due to poor metabolism. Your metabolism is determined by measuring the amount of oxygen used by your body over a specific time frame. When his evaluation is made at rest, it is called the basal metabolic rate (BMR). If you suspect thyroid illness, I'd check it. There are standardized charts all over the Internet. You can check your BMR, but remember, the numbers don't matter a whole lot, it's how you feel, are you thyroid sick, or are you thyroid healthy?! Bear in mind that your BMR is not a hard and fast number, it could be increased with stimulants, living with chronic stress, taking thyroid medicine.

Chapter 11

Depression

There's a connection between low thyroid and depression as well as bipolar disease. Due to poor testing, it rarely gets treated with thyroid medicine. According to the *National Institute of Mental Health*, 9.5% of the US population has a mood disorder and 18% of the US population suffers from anxiety disorders. In my evaluation, if you have depression or bipolar disease, you should be given a trial of thyroid medicine, along with nutrients known to balance neurotransmitters, or adrenal adaptogens. Instead of these things, you get a lifelong prescription for a prescription antidepressant. How do I know this?

The largest study ever done on depression was called the STAR*D trial, and yes the asterisk that appears there is supposed to be there, it is not a typo. The goal of the trial was to compare the effectiveness of depression treatments in people who had major depressive disorders and it was the largest and longest study ever conducted to evaluate depression treatment!

As a pharmacist, we see over 66% of people fail to respond to antidepressant drugs or have side effects severe enough to discontinue use. Of those who do respond to traditional anti-depressant drug therapy, over half will relapse within one year. The STAR*D trial found that T3 medication was effective when other medications were not! Did you catch that, the thyroid worked when the drugs did not! The medications the researchers compared were sertraline (Zoloft), venlafaxine (Effexor), bupro-pion (Wellbutrin) and citalopram (Celexa). The T3 medicine was 50% more effective than certain medications, even with little doses. Patients in the trial tended to lose weight and have more energy.

People with depression are almost always low in thyroid hor-mone, but are prescribed antidepressant drugs instead. You will chase your tail. The risk of bone loss is two to three times higher if you take an SSRI antidepressant, so I really want you to think twice about whether you need that type of drug, as opposed to natural thyroid replacement.

Mood Swings and Bipolar Disease

Thyroid disease often includes mood swings, usually anxiety or irritability but it could be so severe that you are misdiagnosed with bipolar disease and given lithium. Some of you might do better on thyroid medicine.

Researchers evaluated 160 treatment-resistant bipolar patients, that means they are the toughest patients to treat because they don't respond very well to standard bipolar medications. The group they looked at were super tough, the ones who had not responded to an average 14 medications! Imagine the years of suffering for them. I have so much compassion. You can almost guess where I'm going now can't you?! The researchers put these people on T3 medication, regardless of their so-called "normal" TSH value (because it is almost always normal), and 80% of them responded favorably with a reduction in symptoms, and 30% of had complete resolution! With the availability of T3, and other thyroid medications, I see a viable, safe, inexpensive and effective method to help people who are suffering with depression, unstable mood and bipolar disorder.

There was another interesting study where participants had been admitted to an endocrinology outpatient clinic. The group consisted of 51 Hashimoto's thyroiditis patients, 45 patients with goiter (swollen thyroid gland), and 68 control subjects who had no thyroid disease. All participants were assessed for psychiatric disorders which were determined using the "Structured Clinical Interview for DSM-IV." The researchers also used Beck Depression Inventory and Beck Anxiety Inventory with the participants who were diagnosed with a psychiatric disorder.

After analysis of data, the researchers found a statistically significant difference among the three groups in terms of major depression and anxiety. In the Hashimoto's thyroiditis group, the prevalence of depression and panic disorder was significantly higher than that in the control group. However, in the goiter group, mood or depression disorders and anxiety disorders were found to be just as common in comparison to the control group. There was no significant difference found between the Hashimoto's thyroiditis and goiter participants.

The researchers concluded that Hashimoto's thyroiditis patients and goiter patients have an increase predisposition to major depression and anxiety disorders. The researchers suggest that thyroid autoimmunity and other thyroid pathologies should be investigated in depression and anxiety patients with chronic and treatment-resistant complaints. I suggest if you have emotional disorders you test yourself properly to rule out Hashimoto's disease before going on life-long medications like antidepressants, sedatives, psychotropics or mood balancers (lithium). If you have depression or anxiety disorder, you could try some thyroid medication and see how you respond. It beats trying to treat the symptoms with addictive sedatives, sleep aids and antidepressants which don't work for thyroid anyway. Finding the underlying cause will be the answer to your prayers.

Will Synthroid work for you if you have anxiety, depression or bipolar? I doubt it. You see, T4 drugs rarely work for those conditions. NDT (which is combined T4 with T3) works a little better, and T3 works the best with these types of psychiatric conditions. It gets a little complicated, but I want you to know that some people with depression have a genetic snp (a mutation in their DNA) that hinders their ability to transport thyroid hormone into the cell, so they are thyroid sick. In other words, some of you with depression will never ever respond to anti-depressants (or T4 medications) because neither one of those treatments goes into your cells (due to your genetic situation). In this case, T3 drugs are ideal, they slide inside and give your starving cells the bioactive thyroid hormone needed.

I urge you to find a good doctor that will dig deep for you, because if you have depression, your labs look okay to an untrained eye. So you may have normal T4 (or even high), and you might have normal TSH (or even low), so you look "normal" or possibly hyperthyroid to an uneducated physician, but if you dig a little deeper, and take other tests you will likely come up with low levels of "Free T3" and/or high levels of "rT3" or reverse T3. This is the way you can prove you have thyroid resistance, or what I call "thyroid sick" and it's also proof to put you on medication.

This point is huge because millions of people have depression, and the market for the drugs to treat it is in the billions. I'm saying that with depression you may see, relatively normal labs, but it's only because they are not testing Free T3 and rT3 which are often out of normal range. This occurs because you don't transport the T4 into the cell where it gets converted to T3. So you have what is termed thyroid resistance, another way to say that is cellular hypothyroidism, or what I've been calling "thyroid sick" throughout my book. Craving more science? If so, keep reading my next part, otherwise, you have my blessings to skip to the next chapter.

Craving More Science?

This next section is weighted with some science, so if you don't like that please just go on to the next chapter. Otherwise, nerds all aboard! Many things can suppress your TSH causing it to look normal (or even low), which then causes your doctor to believe you are thyroid healthy which is a big mistake. Things that suppress TSH include cortisol from stress, inflammatory cytokines from pain or foods you eat, high prolactin, shifts in neurotransmitters like low serotonin, low dopamine, and low MSH (melanocyte stimulating hormone). So your Free T3 is usually low, rT3 is elevated, it's usually greater than 16 (or 160 depending on the units in which it is reported) and the TSH and T4 are "normal" as a general rule. The overall picture is that your thyroid situation looks fine, but it's not. No antidepressant corrects that, only thyroid medication, proper diet and supplements.

What Is MSH?

You've probably never heard of that, but I specialize in educating you to look at markers that are unconventional. MSH stands for alpha melanocyte stimulating hormone and is abbreviated as αMSH. It's a good thing, you want it around because this hormone is anti-inflammatory, it makes you feel good by helping release endorphins. It controls the release of your sleep hormone, melatonin. It is made in response to leptin, your satiety hormone, the one that says "I feel full." Most people blame obesity and diabetes to overeating but that is old school thinking. Our obesity and diabetes epidemic is really due to damage of MSH and leptin hormones.

MSH deficiencies are tied to chronic fatigue, lots of pain and non-restful sleep (or terrible insomnia for that matter). When MSH is low you will have to pee frequently, and you'll be thirsty all the time (similar to diabetes). You will also be sensitive to electrical shocks, as in neuropathy, or facial pain, or trigeminal neuralgia. Read more about that in my other book, Headache Free, sold at Amazon and my website.

Any illness, including thyroid problems, especially Hashimoto's or Graves' disease will cause the production of inflammation chemicals, and that can cause the MSH deficiency. So you have to address the underlying problem that causes the illness, often an infection, toxins, poisonous antibiotics, biotoxin, mold, fungus, parasite, or food antigen. Refer to Table 4 Thyroid Bombs in Chapter 3, *Thyroid on Fire* to see if you're exposed to, or eating one!

Addressing the underlying problem becomes a challenge if you've had chronic Lyme a long time, or some other undiagnosed illness or food allergy, the hypothalamus takes a hit, the MSH goes down and sometimes it dwindles to nothing. That's about the time you get prescribed Neurontin, Xanax, Ambien or some other drug cocktail to reduce nerve pain, help you relax and help you sleep. There are currently no ways to inject or give you MSH but I will keep you posted if something comes up to help you, there's a huge market for people who are MSH deficient. This biomarker is testable by Quest Labs and others using a blood sample. You can also search research articles on MSH if you go to *Pubmed.com*.

Chapter 12

Heart Disease and High Cholesterol

We normally associate thyroid hormone with weight, mood, metabolism and temperature regulation, but it's critical for the cardiovascular system because it protects your heart and blood vessels. Symptoms of heart problems that go hand-in-hand with thyroid disease include the following:

Bradycardia—on average 10 to 20 beats per minute (slower)
Shortness of breath with little exertion
High blood pressure due to hardening of the arteries
Edema—swollen hands or feet
Chest pain and pressure or angina
Cholesterol abnormalities
Heartbeat irregularities

While the symptoms above can occur in anyone with heart disease, they are often more pronounced in a person with low thyroid. A landmark study from about 15 years ago proved that normal to low thyroid levels raise heart disease risk in women. The shocking part of this study, called the Rotterdam Study (year 2000), was that low thyroid levels were more of a risk factor for heart attack than high cholesterol, smoking, high blood pressure and diabetes. It could contribute to 60% of heart attacks! That information is probably mind blowing because I bet most women with high cholesterol are given statin cholesterol drugs, and I'm saying that they should be tested correctly for hypothyroidism and given a trial course of thyroid medication instead. The study showed that your thyroid levels matters more than your cholesterol. I doubt T4 drugs will work well in this case.

The study found that women with low thyroid levels experienced a significantly higher risk for atherosclerosis (almost twice the risk compared to normal) and heart attack (up to 3 times higher risk than normal). The researchers said, "In conclusion, we found that subclinical hypothyroidism is highly prevalent in elderly women and is strongly and independently associated with aortic atherosclerosis and myocardial infarction ..."

What If You Have A Heart Attack?

You should definitely have your thyroid levels tested properly, read Chapter 5. It's huge trouble if your rT3 is high! Your risk of dying after a heart attack goes up dramatically if you don't optimize your thyroid hormone levels. The one year mortality rate could be anywhere from 40% to 600% higher! If you are worried now, please get yourself tested because heart attacks are sometime preventable if you take good care of yourself. It's not just low thyroid, it's also excessive amounts. If you have what's called "subclinical hyperthyroidism" and produce extra amounts of thyroid, you're also at higher risk for heart attack. Balance is essential. Knowing that your thyroid hormone plays a role in your cardiovascular system is essential to lowering your risk of heart disease and heart attack.

Holy Moly! Statins May Cause Thyroid Problems

These drugs were shown in a study of 307 patients to lower TSH, causing you to look like you're hyperthyroid. This means that if you're taking thyroid medication along with your statin drug

(Lipitor, Zocor, Pravachol, etc) your doctor may try to reduce your thyroid medications based upon a lab test that is artificially messed up. In other words, you may very well be hypothyroid, but your low TSH test will lead a health care professional to suspect you being hyperthyroid. (Remember, the lower your TSH, the less thyroid medicine you'll get). Because statins may falsely lower your serum TSH without affecting tissue levels of T3 and T4, it's called "pseudohyperthyroidism." Keep this in mind if you're being simultaneously treated for high cholesterol and thyroid disease. As I think about it, statins may be a good unconventional treatment for hyperthyroidism or Graves' disease. You just have to replenish what those drug muggers steal. Statins reduce your body's natural vitamin D, CoQ10 and creatine. You should ask your doctor, but I recommend taking those supplements if you are on a statin drug like Lipitor, Zocor, Pravachol, or others. I suggest approximately 5,000 IU vitamin D, 100 mg CoQ10 and 500–100 mg creatine, with a full glass of water each day. Drink lots of water or that creatine will make you cramp.

Chapter 13

Chronic Pain

Many of you live in chronic pain due to injuries, accidents, infections and antibiotic poisoning. No one should have to live in pain, this is a very important subject to me. I even wrote a book on the topic of one of the most disabling pain syndromes entitled "Headache Free: Relieve Migraine, Tension, Cluster, Menstrual and Lyme Headaches."

Being hypothyroid, or thyroid sick can cause pain in and of itself. It can cause headaches, and it can cause widespread pain throughout the body, sometimes diagnosed as fibromyalgia or chronic fatigue syndrome. According to animal studies, hypothyroidism is known to increase a compound in your body known as "Substance P" which sends the signal to your brain so that you notice pain and think "Ouch!" It's considered a pro-inflammatory chemical that you want less of, not more. When a person has low thyroid, the degree to which they feel pain is increased because of higher levels of this Substance P which make you more sensitive to pain.

The plot thickens because Substance P coexists in your body with the excitatory neurotransmitter glutamate, and those 2 compounds together are pretty nasty in terms of what they do to you. Normal physiological levels are fine, but in excess it's nasty. You really want to tame those beasts somehow, because high levels of Substance P and glutamate equal high anxiety, major depression, nausea or vomiting, heightened sensitivity to pain, respiratory rhythm disturbances, insomnia, post-traumatic stress disorder (PTSD) and Raynaud's phenomena. You can understand now why it's important to optimize thyroid function because if you don't, you get all these loose cannons in your body that contribute to these other disorders.

The following pain syndromes are commonly associated with low levels of thyroid hormone:

Muscle aches and weakness
Stiffness of the joints (especially hips, shoulders, knees)
Swollen knee joints
Carpal tunnel syndrome
Neuropathy (numbness, burning, tingling)

Certain medications like opiate analgesics (oxycodone, hydro-codone) as well as gabapentin (Neurontin) and pregabalin (Lyrica) reduce Substance P. Natural remedies that reduce Substance P include ginger root, capsaicin, Bromelain from pineapples, quercetin, corydalis and curcumin.

Analgesics and Thyroid Medicine

As a pharmacist for more than 2 decades, I've noticed that there's a common prescription combination that is dispensed. It's your medication for thyroid and your medication for pain. The pain pills vary, but often it is for something like Neurontin, Lyrica, Vicodin, Percocet or a few others. This says to me that low thyroid and pain go together. You may be taking ibuprofen (Advil, Motrin) or naproxen (Aleve) every day, these are sold over-the-counter. Autoimmune thyroid disease (such as Hashimoto's) will make your pain syndrome even worse. The pain and the thyroid disease are driven by one thing, the same thing. It's high amounts of pro-inflammatory cytokines. You have to bring those pain-causing chemicals down and in doing so, you treat both conditions at once.

This is why curcumin, resveratrol and green tea are so useful for some of you. I covered this extensively in my headache book, and the options I offered there could easily apply to any pain syndrome, not just headaches.

The Thyroid Connection to Pain

The big secret is that chronic pain will significantly cause a reduction in tissue T3, without even altering your TSH! So if your doctor uses the standard method of thyroid testing (which is TSH and T4 levels) it will appear normal, but it is anything but! You could be dismissed with a normal thyroid when you're thyroid sick. Do you live in chronic pain? If the answer is yes, you may need more thyroid hormone, a trial for 14 days would show whether or not you were going to respond well. I'm telling you that your labs will reflect a normal TSH causing you to be dismissed with a normal thyroid, but if more testing were to be done it would likely show a low level of tissue T3. The way to find out is to have 2 tests done on your next blood draw: Free T3 and Reverse T3 (rT3). You then take the ratio of those two (Free T3 divided by rT3) and it should be > 2 for you to feel better. I've made it very easy for you by uploading a conversion tool that automatically converts your units so in 10 seconds, you're done. I've named it "Easy Thyroid Lab Converter" and it's posted at both of my websites, *www.ScriptEssentials.com/ThyroidConverter* and *www.Suzy-Cohen.com/ThyroidConverter*. In addition to this Free T3/rT3 ratio, it's good to evaluate your antibody levels to see if your thyroid is on fire.

Medications for Pain Complicate Things

My goal for this chapter is to help you realize that taking thyroid medication along with your pain medication could work well. I think the combination will do you much better than either medication alone. I'm never going to tell you to suffer, and go without pain medicine but I need to teach you something else that is important: *Pain medications prevent activation of your thyroid hormone.* Specifically, some of these drugs suppress the conversion of T4 to T3 which adds to your hypothyroid condition.

Opiate analgesics (Percocet, Morphine, Vicodin, etc) are useful and effective at alleviating pain but I want your physician to take even better care of you by trying some thyroid hormone medication or supplements. I think your response will be better than what you get now. The use of pain pills (without thyroid replacement) won't be helpful in the long run.

Chronic pain significantly suppresses D1, and stimulates D2, resulting in a reduction of tissue T3 but normal to higher thyroid levels in the brain. That may sound complicated to you, but I've included that information for your doctor's benefit. You can read about D1 and D2 enzymes on page 23 in the section entitled, The "D" Enzymes. It just means your labs look superb but you feel awful. You (and every achy bone in your body) will be sent home without adequate treatment unless you know this. Your tissues are starving for thyroid hormone, hence you are thyroid sick but your labs look relatively "normal" unless certain tests are conducted (I'll tell you in a minute). The opiate analgesics action on thyroid hormone will exacerbate depression and fatigue commonly seen with chronic pain syndromes.

Do you understand now, why I keep saying that the TSH doesn't matter, and yet this is the standard blood test used for patients who are suspected of having thyroid disorders. It's the standard of practice so you can't be mad at your doctor, you just have to empower yourself with this kind of information, then ask for correct testing because they are not taught this in school, and they are not nerds like me so they don't study for a living in order to write books on health. They don't devote years of their life to studying thyroid, and they haven't necessarily suffered with low thyroid either. You can ask your doctor to get you tested, and you can also order tests directly to your home from a page I've set up to simplify things, *www.DirectLabs.com/SuzyCohen.*

Should You Take Your Pain Medicine?

Yes of course. By no means am I suggesting you go without pain pills, I'm a huge advocate for anything that relieves pain for you. Over time, once your thyroid hormone is optimized, you may find that you need lower and lower dosages of your pain pills. That would be delightful to hear. It would mean you were living thyroid healthy, just like the title of my book. I'm teaching you about this controversial subject so that you will know to ask your doctor for adequate thyroid medication even if you already take pain pills.

There are many excellent pain specialists who understand thyroid disease well enough to understand everything you have just read and then some. I've simplified it. Your physician may recommend T3 medications, or combination T4/T3 (like Armour Thyroid or Thyrolar and others) despite that normal TSH. The only drug that I would not recommend (because it will not work well) is a pure T4 drug. Remember, the problem with those medications is that you can't convert T4 to T3 very well, and you need T3 inside the cell. The T4 drugs won't be ideal for you if you have chronic pain.

If you have to take opiate analgesics, bear in mind these can be very constipating, and that is already a problem in people with thyroid disease. You may want to include fiber from fruits and vegetables, hemp seed, chia seeds or rice cereal. You can also buy psyllium husk fiber supplements and powders. Probiotics are important for people with constipation and low thyroid so these are a must!

Thyroid Healthy Tip

Your mattress! Flame retardants commonly found in your bed are accumulating in peoples bodies and these compounds can block thyroid (Toxological Sciences 2000).

Chapter 14

Iron Deficiency and Chronic Fatigue

L ow iron leads to chronic fatigue, it is the hallmark symptom. But that said, not all fatigue is related to iron deficiency. Still, when you talk about thyroid illness, you must talk about low iron too, because these 2 conditions often go hand in hand.

Iron helps you make a protein called hemoglobin, which acts like a tow truck and lugs oxygen all over the body. As humans, we can stash some iron away in the form called "ferritin" until it's needed. Iron deficiency includes feeling cold, irritable, depressed or having a hard time concentrating. Having pale lips, or pale skin and a sore tongue are dead giveaways. Brittle nails and frequent infections may also alert you to low iron. When I dealt with this problem, my heart would beat faster with very little exertion.

If you drink a lot of dark grape juice or red wine you may need additional iron. Also, if you have heavy menstrual cycles you are losing a lot more blood, so I'd recommend testing yourself for iron deficiency. Finally, if you are low in digestive acid, you will not fully extract your iron from your meals and may need a little help, in the form of "betaine with pepsin."

Cold All The Time?

If you're low in iron, you will feel cold all the time. It could be low thyroid and it could be low iron. The *American Journal of Clinical Nutrition* published a study that investigated the relationship between iron-deficiency anemia and our ability to warm up after a cold water bath. Ten women with iron-deficiency anemia, 8 women with depleted iron stores (non- anemic), and 12 control women participated in this study. All of the women had similar body fat percentages and were exposed to a cold water bath of 28 degrees C for 100 minutes. The researchers found the anemic women to have significantly lower body temperatures and T3 and T4 concentrations than the control participants at the base-line and after the cold water bath exposure.

The second phase of this study gave the iron deficient women ferrous sulfate, an iron supplement for 12 weeks. The control group got nothing. Then they all jumped back into the cold water bath, several times in fact! Long story short, the researchers were able to prove that once the iron levels were increased (but not to normal) the T3 and T4 levels improved, as did their ability to stay warmer during the horrid cold baths which you couldn't pay me to take. The point is that if you're low in iron, your thyroid hormone isn't going to work for you, and you'll be more prone to cold sensitivity.

The research tells me that thyroid-hormone metabolism is significantly affected in people with iron-deficient anemia. I can tell you first hand because I lived it, my ferritin was 8 (it should be between 70 and 90!) and I had some symptoms of thyroid disease, mainly profound fatigue, brittle nails that didn't grow very fast, dry skin, especially my heels and poor concentration. (Read Chapter 23). Now, years later with optimal thyroid levels I feel really good. I still have the dry skin though, which I rationalize to living in a desert. I buy lotion. It's a small price to pay for living in the 'screen saver' it's just so pretty here in Colorado!

Now, the big point here is that if you have low iron (or low ferritin levels), you cannot activate your thyroid hormone T4 to T3. This means you have poor conversion. On a lab, your TSH may appear fine, and your T4 might be normal too, or perhaps even elevated (because it's not converting to T3). One way to help yourself here is to take a little iron (iron bisglycinate is a good brand) along with a little iodine and see if you start feeling better. This should only be done with your doctor's permission.

Since I think with a broad paintbrush, I'd like you to have as many options as possible so, I will now mention another tip I learned from Dr. Kent Holtorf (holtorfmed.com). For chronic, stubborn low ferritin, he mentions low dose heparin, which is a blood thinner that you take by subcutaneous injection. This is commonly given in IVs when you go to the hospital, but we are talking about low doses. When we say "low dose" we mean it, because heparin can be dangerous in high doses causing internal hemorrhage. Heparin is an anticoagulant and it shuttles your red blood cells more efficiently, oxygenating your whole body in a manner that doesn't normally occur when you're really iron deficient. I'd consider this if your ferritin drops below 10.

Why Are You Pale?

Thyroid dilates blood vessels, so when it's low you have less blood flow to the skin and tend to be pale. You can also be pale if your iron is low, meaning you have anemia.

Chapter 15

PMS, Pregnancy and Infertility

I believe every single woman, at some point in her life, becomes hypothyroid to a certain degree. It's because of the female hormones becoming imbalanced as you go through your menstrual cycles. Here comes a little known secret, and it holds the connection between female hormones and thyroid. We know that women are dramatically more likely to have thyroid disease. The secret is this: With declining hormones, females generate more and more of a protein called "thyroid binding globulin" or TBG which binds up your active T3 making it unusable to your cells!

Your symptoms are not in your head, and I'm sorry that physicians don't believe you. You may even be made to feel like a hypochondriac but you are not! When you're handed an antidepressant, it's the same as saying, "I don't believe you, this is all in your head." You can fire an insensitive doctor you know, and find a respectful doctor that believes you and cares about helping you. You do have that power.

Female hormones play an essential role in thyroid health. If you're thyroid is low it will cause more symptoms of premenstrual syndrome or PMS. It can affect your ability to get pregnant, and carry your baby. Thyroid hormone imbalances cause menopausal symptoms too. Balancing your hormones is essential. No matter how much thyroid medication you take, if your hormones are imbalanced, you're not going to respond well. The more TBG you make the more thyroid sick you are. You can measure the TBG with a blood test.

Surges of estrogen which you get from 'The Pill' or from erratic fluctuations during peri-menopause can make your symptoms worse. As the estrogen fluctuates, it puts your immune system on red alert, and makes it more sensitive to everything. In a menopausal or peri-menopausal woman, this can cause more furious hot flashes and insomnia, anxiety and irritability.

If you have Hashimoto's disease, and most people with low thyroid do have the autoimmune component to their thyroid disease (diagnosed or not), then estrogen surges will make you feel worse at a certain time of the month. Count on it every month! The estrogen surge causes an increase in TBG as I explained earlier in this chapter, and it makes your active thyroid hormone unusable to you. Your cells are starving for thyroid, even if your TSH is normal. Pregnancy will affect hormones too. In fact there's a connection to pregnancy and Hashimoto's disease. At a certain time during your pregnancy, the hormone fluctuations can fire up your Hashimoto's disease because of changes in your immune cells. After you give birth, you may also feel worse. This is not a hard fast rule, I just want you to know that hormonal shifts during and after pregnancy can cause flares.

Where Is Your Hair Loss?

Just on top? That's probably low estrogen
Male pattern? Think high DHT (dihydrotestosterone)
All over? It's likely low thyroid

'The Pill' Can Make You Sleepy

Certain conditions like stress cause you to make more rT3. The reason for that is because stress increases cortisol, your stress hormone. Extremely high cortisol is referred to as Cushing's syndrome. When your cortisol is high it speeds up conversion of T4 to rT3 by affecting certain enzymes. You don't want a lot of rT3, it sends you into hibernation mode. RT3 is a metabolite of T4 (thyroxine). Typically, when T4 loses an atom of iodine, it becomes triiodothyronine (T3), the active thyroid hormone. But in some cases, the body conserves energy by converting the T4 instead into RT3, an inactive form of T3 that is incapable of delivering oxygen and energy to the cells, as T3 would. Elevated levels of rT3 (and therefore low thyroid hormone) is more predictive of death than high cholesterol. Has anyone informed you of this? Has your rT3 been evaluated? Or are you just one of millions of people told you're okay and let's "wait and see" what happens. Wait for what? A heart attack? There's a higher risk of cardiovascular disease associated with 'The Pill.'

You want real, bioactive T3 to wake you up. If you take pure T4 drugs like Levothyroxine you also see increased conversion to sleepy rT3. Ladies, here's something to stun you. If you take estrogen-containing medications such as birth control pills, shots or patches, you'll make more rT3. If you take menopause medications with synthetic estrogens you may also make more rT3. If you have estrogen dominance (aka progesterone deficiency), or iron deficiency (as in low ferritin) the same situation occurs. You become thyroid sick despite normal thyroid tests which only look for classic "hypothyroidism."

Birth control is also used in young teenagers to treat acne. The high estrogen from this, along with the nutrient depletions from the pill (zinc, magnesium, folate and tyrosine) will make you thyroid sick over time. Did you just say "Ah ha!" How are you supposed to lose weight and look beautiful when your hormones are imbalanced and your cells are starving for nutrients? This is a disadvantage to taking oral contraception, but now that you know you can restore lost nutrients, or consider another method of contraception.

'The Pill' causes your SHBG (sex hormone binding globulin) to go up dramatically, and stay up even if you discontinue it. You can measure SHBG with a blood test very easily. Mind blowing information now: Elevations in SHBG lower testosterone, your sex drive hormone! This also means you need more thyroid hormone medication because low testosterone means reduced activation to T3. So when you take 'The Pill', you will lose your sex drive and eventually require thyroid medicine. Going off 'The Pill' can restore libido in some cases.

Plastic Water Bottles Too?

Fake dangerous estrogens termed "xenoestrogens" and heavy metals increase your levels of sleepy rT3. There are many harmful chemicals in commercial cosmetics, household cleaners, foods and even our tap water. Plastic bottles that contain Bisphenol A (BPA) are another common example of how you can ingest chemicals that block thyroid receptors with rT3, so thyroid hormone never gets into the cell (thyroid sick).

What's a girl to do?! You can either unblock the receptor and knock the rT3 off (so thyroid hormone can get in), or you can take a different type of thyroid medicine. Any savvy endocrinologist can correct this situation if it's recognized. That's the big deal, recognition. You see, the TSH will often remain normal even though BPA, or some other xenoestrogen has blocked the thyroid receptor. They are termed "endocrine disrupters" if you want to look it up.

Flame retardants in your mattress and pesticides sprayed in your home do the same awful thing. Pesticides have estrogen, so I'd avoid commercial foods and buy organic when possible. As for heavy metals, the list is long including cadmium from smoking, mercury, thimerosol, seafood (especially tuna and sea bass), and pollutants. All of these adversely impact your thyroid hormone by blocking the thyroid receptor or preventing activation of T4.

More specifically, these chemicals may drive the conversion of T4 to rT3 (inactive) instead of T3 (active) by disrupting enzymes.

Do You Have Fertility Issues?

There are more than 6.1 million women affected with infertility, and many pay a lot of money for in vitro fertilization. I wonder how many women could have conceived if their thyroid function was optimized? I know lots of women who optimized thyroid hormone and ultimately got pregnant. Today, their children are almost all grown and they are thankful to the doctor who recognized their hypothyroid state and corrected it. If your dream is to have a baby, and you can't, I recommend you read this entire book and have your thyroid problems addressed correctly. Iodine deficiency is crucial for women who want to become pregnant or nurse their infants. Iodine deficiency in the pregnant woman has been associated with miscarriages, stillbirth, preterm delivery, and congenital abnormalities in the babies. Children of mothers with severe iodine deficiency during pregnancy can have mental retardation and problems with growth, hearing, and speech. In the most severe form, hypothyroidism in mother can result in cretinism (a syndrome characterized by permanent brain damage, mental retardation, deaf mutism, spasticity, and short stature). This is not as frequently seen in the United States as it is in other countries. The point is have your iodine levels evaluated with an overnight urine sample to find out if you need this natural mineral. Restoring iodine (which creates thyroid hormone) is so much simpler and cheaper than fertility treatments.

I asked my friend Dana Trentini about the subject of pregnancy and thyroid disease. She is the founder of "Hypothyroid Mom" the mission of which is to fight for universal thyroid screening in pregnancy. According to Dana, "Every woman planning to conceive, and every woman currently pregnant, should have a complete thyroid test that includes markers such as TSH, Free T4, Free T3,

Reverse T3, and thyroid antibodies. Research reveals the dangers of thyroid disease (specifically deficiency of thyroid) in pregnancy including miscarriage, still birth, infertility, maternal anemia, pre-eclampsia, placental abruption, postpartum hemorrhage, premature delivery, low birth weight and deficits in intellectual development in infants." Isn't that just amazing?! It is a big clue for lots of ladies who have dealt with these problems. Dana writes Hypothyroid Mom in memory of the unborn baby she lost to hypothyroidism. You can learn more about her, and sign up for her newsletter at *www.HypothyroidMom.*

Low Thyroid Causes Miscarriages

The statistics make no mistake, miscarriage is the leading compli-cation of pregnancy. It is estimated that one in five pregnancies end in a miscarriage. I wonder how often this heartbreaking loss is due to undiagnosed thyroid conditions, specifically higher levels of antibodies against the thyroid. The most popular one tested is the TPO antibody, abbreviated like this, TPOAb. Research suggests that pregnant women have a higher risk of miscarriage if their TPO antibodies are elevated and they often are in hypothyroidism. You usually get the diagnosis of Hashimoto's when your TPOAb are high.

Researchers conducted a study measuring TPOAb in 118 women who had experienced a miscarriage and had never birthed a live born child. They compared this to 162 women who had two or more live births and never miscarried.

The data found women who had suffered one or more mis-carriages had higher antibody levels than those in the control group (no miscarriages). This study confirmed the association between miscarriage and increased TPO antibodies, what I refer to as thyroid on fire! Based upon this research, I highly recommend you test your blood for levels of TPO antibodies, as well as the other antibodies for autoimmune thyroid disease, before getting pregnant, and especially if you have a history of miscarriage. It may uncover the clue to why you are not carrying your baby full term. I really want to get your love notes for this tidbit of information. Infertility and miscarriages are really common in women with undiagnosed thyroid disease.

PMS Gets Worse With Low Thyroid

A study to determine the prevalence of hypothyroidism in patients with benign breast cysts found that 23 percent of the women tested had undiagnosed hypothyroidism. Symptoms of fibrocystic breast disease were alleviated in 83 percent of the hypothyroid females with just the use of T4 (thyroxin) hormone replacement. (*World Journal of Surgery*, July 2009)

Studies show that heavy menstrual flow and premenstrual syndrome (PMS) is often related to low thyroid. When you treat the low thyroid levels, your cycles could get better. PMS could also be tied to high estrogen. Your doctor can do proper testing to help you find out if you have either one of these conditions. There are two tests I recommend, which your physician can order for you. Any physician can order this test, but some of you are going to meet with resistance when you ask. For that reason, I've arranged for you to buy lab tests directly from my affiliate link (thus taking the kink out for you). They sell labs direct to consumer, go to *www.DirectLabs.com/SuzyCohen* and the two tests I recommend are:

1. Basic Female Profile by Genova
2. Complete Thyroid Panel plus Thyroid Antibodies

There's a connection between premenstrual syndrome (PMS) and thyroid disorders. A study published in the *New England Journal of Medicine* investigated the incidence of hypothyroidism in women with PMS. This was a well-designed study that included all sorts of thyroid evaluations and tests.

The researchers found that 94 of 100 ladies with PMS had low thyroid compared to 0 of the women who had easy periods. Zero!

The clincher is that 65% of hypothyroid women had thyroid labs come back with numbers in the so-called "normal" range. They were missed by the TSH test which I keep telling you is not my favorite test, and here's another reason why, right?! This is the important part though, the women with PMS enjoyed complete relief of their symptoms once they took thyroid hormone replacement drugs, even though their standard TSH blood tests were "normal." So basically, they were treated regardless of their "normal" labs and their PMS got better. I am pretty sure many of you reading my book have also fallen through the cracks.

Another study published in the *American Journal of Psychiatry* also investigated thyroid function in women with PMS. Guess what? The researchers showed that 7 of 10 women with PMS were thyroid sick despite having normal TSH levels, on their conventional blood test. Let me take off my white pharmacy coat and talk to you like my soul sister, as if we were chatting over a carrot juice. I'd lean over and say it this way, "The TSH blood tests suck! Don't rely on them to help you lose weight, look beautiful or live the life you imagine." Follow the "Script" I offer in Chapter 24, *Live Thyroid Healthy*.

Help for PMS and Peri-Menopausal Symptoms

Magnesium. If you cry easily or feel irritable and moody, this is great. It's also wonderful for fibromyalgia pain and for leg cramps. Magnesium is essential to you making energy! You can't make ATP without it. It's depleted from your body by 100s of medications as well as antacids, acid blockers and birth control. You can try a little bit of magnesium glycinate, malate or citrate, about 200-300 mg once or twice daily.

Green tea. It is meditation in a teacup because it contains a sub-stance that's instantly calming called L-theanine. Careful though, studies are decidedly mixed! In the August 2010 issue of *Human and Experimental Toxicology* green tea (when compared to black tea) caused a dramatic reduction in thyroid hormones T3 and T4. The TSH (thyroid stimulating hormone), was increased with green tea, indicating that it adversely affects the thyroid gland. Green tea may also cause slight enlargement of the thyroid gland. The jury is out on green tea and thyroid health, some say it's wonderful, others say to avoid. You just have to track your symptoms.

Rhodiola rosea. The Siberian herb is calming, about 50-100 mg twice daily. Capsules or liquid extract are best.

St. John's Wort. It helps if you get a little moody with your periods, because it is a natural mood stabilizer. It's helpful for emotional, as well as some physical symptoms of PMS. St. John's wort interacts with oral contraception and many other drugs so make sure your practitioner approves before you take it.

5-hydroxytryptophan (5-HTP). This is a precursor to serotonin, a happy brain chemical. It's sold as a supplement.

Flax Seed. Sprinkle ground up flax seeds on your food. They help curtail the effects of excessive estrogens in the body that you get from "The Pill" or from drinking out of plastic water bottles.

I3C or DIM. Diindolylmethane is a component of I3C, also sold at health food stores and online. DIM is a naturally occurring phytonutrient that is found in the cruciferous vegetables broccoli, Brussels sprouts, cabbage, and kale. Why 2 supplements? In order for you to convert IC3 to DIM in your body, there has to be adequate stomach acid. People over 40 years old, produce significantly less stomach acid. DIM may be a better choice if you are over 40 years old. This supplement processes estrogen in a way that lowers harmful by-products. This goes a long way in shrinking fibroids, easing heavy periods and reducing cramps.

Thyroid or Ritalin?

Parents of children with "attention deficit" are at a loss for what to do. They mean well and often administer strong prescription drugs to help with ADD or ADHD. There is research to show that giving natural thyroid hormone medications, specifically T3, can be very effective, without the side effects of Ritalin, Adderall and Concerta. Testing your child correctly is imperative so please read Chapter 5, *The Best Lab Tests.*

I interviewed patient advocate Mary Shomon, who is the New York Times best-selling author of "Thyroid Diet Revolution." She had lots to say about getting thyroid healthy and asked me to share this with you.

The number one thing a thyroid patient can do to live and feel well is to be informed. We assume our doctors will tell us the basics, for example, how a high to normal TSH may be a sign of hypothyroidism, or that you can have significant thyroid symptoms despite a normal TSH test result when you have Hashimoto's disease. We assume they'll tell us that you shouldn't take your thyroid medication at the same time as iron or calcium, and that T3 or natural thyroid might work better for us than Synthroid. We assume they'll inform us that a gluten-free diet could actually "cure" some cases of hypothyroidism. Unfortunately, for the most part, they don't tell us these basics so it's really up to thyroid patients to become informed, ask questions, and find knowledgeable experts and doctors to partner with for the best care.

You can learn more about Mary Shomon at:
www.Thyroid-Info.com

Chapter 16

Hashimoto's Disease

You can have symptoms for years and never know. You can get all kinds of diagnoses for 15 diseases, but it just might be one thing, Hashimoto's. It's sad that doctors say this condition is rare, because it really isn't. It's epidemic, it is so terribly misdiagnosed. You may suffer for years before you are correctly diagnosed. Hashi's is responsible for upwards of 80% of every case of hypothyroidism. You may have it yourself. Most doctors just don't know how to test for it because the immunity and cytokine tests, and classic antibody tests are not that telling. One day, science will catch up and we will find that most cases of thyroid disease are tied to autoimmune dysfunction.

It's an autoimmune disease where your own immune system attacks your tissue. Not everyone gets the autoimmune version, but most people, about 80% with thyroid disease have some degree of autoimmune attack. You may be referring to your condition as "chronic thyroiditis" or Hashi's. There are many theories, one of which is molecular mimicry where the immune system recognizes a germ and builds antibodies to it. But the parts of this germ (proteins in it) looks similar to a gland or organ. It's a case of mistaken identity. Your nerve fibers get attacked in the autoimmune condition called multiple sclerosis, your joints in the case of rheumatoid arthritis. With Hashimoto's it's your thyroid gland.

Getting diagnosed is the key, so many of you have fallen through the cracks. In the initial stages of Hashimoto's there are swings in thyroid hormone, it goes up and down, which is known as Hashitoxicosis. Your mood will swing wildly too, and many Hashi sufferers get misdiagnosed with bipolar disease. Then, they are prescribed medications such as carbamazepine or others which are strong 'drug muggers' of nutrients. What happens next looks just like hypothyroidism because the drugs cause your body to develop dry skin, constipation, hair loss, insomnia and more. Read Chapter 23, *Solutions for Thyroid Symptoms,* to get help with some of these common thyroid symptoms.

Getting diagnosed correctly is crucial and I worry how many of you with "bipolar disease" really had Hashimoto's instead. No amount of lithium or carbamazepine will correct Hashi symptoms, although it does stabilize mood.

Thyroid antibody testing is not routine, especially in younger women, or in women that don't have classic thyroid symptoms so it's your job to ask for these tests. Even testing is sketchy. It's common to have just the TPO enzyme antibodies tracked in Hashimoto's disease as a measure of progress, but there are several others that should be evaluated. Read Chapter 5, *The Best Lab Tests.*

Most cases of hypothyroidism are Hashimoto's, but not all. There has to be the perfect storm. You have to have certain genes causing a predisposition, and then the trigger (like a food allergy, or infection). You'll also need a leaky gut which most people have. I'm not being sarcastic when I say "leaky gut." Your intestines become permeable, meaning they can't hold their contents correctly, so microscopic food particles slip out and enter your blood stream. Your blood totes these particles and proteins around your body and eventually drops them off in a tissue.

Your immune system does what it's supposed to do, it chases down the foreigner (antigen) in whatever tissue it lodged in, for example, your thyroid gland. It kills the cells that boarding up the foreigner. You can't blame your immune system, it's doing what it's supposed to. You want it to chase out and kill foreigners! The problem is not with your immune system, it's with your leaky gut. So you have to think in terms of locking the doors on your gut! Scientifically, we have to improve intestinal permeability and make it such that the tiny holes in your gut close up and stop leaking. This is why everyone talks about eating better when you have an autoimmune disease. Your eating habits have a direct effect on your Hashi's, in fact any autoimmune disorder. Your thyroid gland is on fire, and to put the fire out you have to reduce antigen load from your gland. You do that by removing food antigens (or killing bacteria if it's related to a pathogen). You should read Chapter 5, *The Best Lab Tests* and learn about zonulin, the molecule responsible for closing up the holes in you leaky gut.

What's the #1 Way to Help Hashi's?

Avoid grains and other food antigens. This helps to bring down your antibodies quickly. You can test for foods you are allergic to with U.S. Biotek labs and others. This halts the progression of Hashimoto's, but of course, supplements are needed to repair the gut lining.

What are food antigens? They can be any food particle that leaks out, and they upset your thyroid gland, and causes the antibodies to rise. You have to determine what it is. For most people, it is dairy or gluten but can also be soy. Soy is actually a very common food antigen and it also is a goitrogen meaning it reduces thyroid hormone production. Avoiding tofu and soy milk can go a long way for Hashi sufferers, and in some cases that's all you have to do. I highly recommend Doug Kaufmann's Phase One Diet, the SCD (specific carbohydrate diet), or the Paleo Diet. These are grain-free diets. One of my friends had very high antibodies (in the 300 range) and I urged her to eat grain-free, and her antibodies fell into the normal range in 8 months.

What's the #2 Way to Help Hashi's?

Get rid of an infection and your life could get better. *What do you mean you don't have one?* You absolutely might and not even know it. We are all loaded with germs. Don't freak out, but there are more germs in us than blood cells. Have you ever had mono? Have you ever had chicken pox? Did you get vaccinated. Do you realize what is on your skin?! Germs. They're everywhere, especially in your mouth and nose.

Do you have reflux disease? Then you might have H. Pylori infection. Another common infection is Lyme disease which you can get from a tick bite that your dog or cat brings into the house. Most people with Lyme have an autoimmune disease and it can look just like Hashimoto's disease! Chronic Lyme (often undetected) is a trigger for all sorts of changes in thyroid hormone. Many people who think they have fibromyalgia or chronic fatigue get tested and find out they actually have Lyme, and they are always hypothyroid. It's too complex to explain here. I talked about Lyme disease more thoroughly in my Headache Free book (available at Amazon) and I've posted articles to my website.

The herpes viruses like cytomegalovirus and EBV (Epstein-Barre virus) are linked to Hashimoto's. I think infections drive many illnesses and cause many people to be misdiagnosed. The body's reaction to biotoxins and infectious bugs is to pump out antibodies and with Hashi's you see an increase in several antibodies, usually TPO or thyroglobulin. As adults we are loaded with toxins and Hashi patients are allergic to many foods and chemicals. It all accumulates. The *Environmental Working Group* reported an average of 232 chemicals found in the cord blood of babies. After birth, babies are often vaccinated and the accumulation continues. Root canals are even responsible for harboring germs in some people. These microorganisms cause autoimmune disorders. You need to know this because treatment for your symptoms doesn't get to the true infectious cause. You can take a "Stimulated

Cytokines" test from Metametrix if you want to get a better picture of infections in your body.

Let's Hear It For The Antibodies

Antibodies are proteins used by your immune system to fight the foreign invaders, usually bacteria, fungus, and viruses. When your immune system sees a threat, it makes an antibody. If it makes an antibody to thyroperoxidase enzyme (TPO), then your thyroid pays the price. These antibodies are detected on a blood test. The lower the number the better for you. If you have your lab results, go get them now. You will see a measurement for TPO antibodies, sometimes abbreviated as "TPOAb."

You may also see thyroglobulin antibodies (TgAb) on your lab test. Measuring this is just as important as TPO antibodies. Again, the lower the number the better. Antibodies can be thought of as soldiers that attack your thyroid gland and kill cells in it. Eventually you will lose your ability to make thyroid hormone if you don't get these soldiers to back off. The reason I'm teaching you about antibodies, is because there's something important for you to understand that your antibodies will be high for many years *before* your TSH blood level becomes abnormal. This is crucial information for you, because some physicians miss the opportunity to test you early on. If you're tested for 'thyroid antibodies' early enough, you'll have years to take care of yourself and head off a Hashi diagnosis.

Now that you know this, you can request the blood test, a 'thyroid antibody' profile and you should ask for it even if you have a normal TSH. Elevated antibodies is your cue that your thyroid is under attack, read Chapter 3, *Thyroid on Fire*.

This tragedy occurs because antibody testing is not done routinely, especially in women under 40. They test your T4 and your TSH as a standard rule, if normal they never do the antibody test!

Antibody testing is particularly important if you have a family history of thyroid disease. If this is elevated you can start to quickly treat yourself, and uncover food antigens (or infections) which drive autoimmune disorders and irritate the heck out of your immune cells. I'm happy if you do them just annually or more often if you're chronically ill. Elevated TPO antibodies means your thyroid is being eaten alive basically. But lab tests aren't always accurate, and sometimes you're told you're okay when you're not because doc is testing your T4 and TSH and if they are "normal" then you're dismissed. In fact, the rate of false negatives are upwards of 40% meaning you could have Hashi's and not know it from your blood test. The rate of false positives are below 3%. This means if your lab shows you are positive, it's probably accurate. In my perfect scenario, I would have you take 2 tests or even 3 to see the trend. The antibodies have a tendency to go up and down, especially at first, so several tests over 6 months, offer a more meaningful trend. After a while of having Hashimoto's, you will settle into a state of permanent hypothyroidism because your gland is destroyed and stops producing thyroxine (T4). Take the antibody tests to detect this early, and be aggressive with your lifestyle and diet to calm the situation.

When it comes to evaluating Hashimoto's, antibodies are not the be-all, end-all. I say that because even your TPO antibodies might be normal because you are Th1 dominant. The discussion of Th1 and Th2 dominance is covered fully in my other book, *Eczema, Itchin' For A Cure*. What In a nutshell, this means your immune system is so frazzled, it can't even produce proper antibodies anymore, so your level is normal on a lab test, (when it should be high), and your thyroid is really on fire despite the "normal" TPO antibodies. If you have all the symptoms of Hashi's and there are clues to prove it, I'd take that diagnosis despite a normal TPO. I know it's confusing. I wish it were black and white, but so many things with thyroid disease are based on your clinical presentation, and your symptoms rather than labs. The labs are only a piece of the puzzle, they're not always right.

Heard of Hashimoto's Encephalopathy?

If you don't know about this complication of hypothyroidism, you are likely to get diagnosed with a seizure disorder, or a stroke. Hashimoto's encephalopathy literally looks like you're having a stroke. The medications used to treat seizures and stroke symptoms do nothing for this type of encephalopathy and a patient could die if misdiagnosed. You need high doses of steroid medications to control this complication, but if you don't know that, you will be treated for a stroke (or seizure) and may not get the help you need in time.

The Best Treatments for Hashimoto's Disease

Selenium supplementation
Low Dose Naltrexone or LDN
Testosterone replacement
Vitamin D3 which regulates the immune system
L-Glutamine because it reestablishes the gut lining
Probiotics because they modulate the gastrointestinal tract
Digestive enzymes, especially dipeptidyl peptidase (DPPIV)

Selenium. This powerful mineral can help you achieve your number one goal which is to suppress antibodies by up to 40%. You cannot make glutathione without selenium in your body. You need glutathione because it is a full-body housekeeper so it detoxifies you. It's incredibly important to your health and well-being. Consider 100 - 200 mcg selenium every day or ask your doctor what's right for you. Too much will give you palpitations.

Low Dose Naltrexone. This is a special compounded prescription drug so it's not sold at regular pharmacies, just compounding ones. Your physician must call it in. Most of the time, it is called in as 1.5mg capsules at first so you can titrate your dosage up until you're taking LDN 4.5mg each night. LDN is made by compounding pharmacies. If it gives you bad dreams, take it during the day. I know you will read not to take it during the day, but I'm saying that it's okay, you should still get some effect without the insomnia or bad dreams that occurs sometimes. You can also try taking it at night, but take a lower dose, like 1.5mg or 3mg. I asked my good friend Julia Schopick to weigh in on LDN. She is the best-selling author of *Honest Medicine, Effective, Time-Tested, Inexpensive Treatments for Life-Threatening Diseases.* "LDN appears to be effective for some diseases that have, at their core, a dysfunctional immune system. It may be helpful for Hashimoto's or Graves' disease even though those conditions have opposite effects on thyroid hormone levels, and the reason is because they are both due to immune dysfunction aimed at the thyroid gland. One interesting side effect that some people mention with LDN is vivid dreams."

Testosterone. Yes, the manly hormone. Some women are too low in this hormone and that reduces T3 activation. In other words, low "T" makes you hypothyroid. We also know normal physiological values of testosterone calm down the antibody attack. Testosterone levels will go dramatically lower in a woman who takes birth control pills or patches. If you have low levels of testosterone, you'll want to bring that hormone up. You can evaluate your testosterone levels with a doctor that knows how to test, usually urine tests. I offer some of these at my affiliate lab site which allows labs to be sold 'direct to consumer.' Just go to, *www.DirectLabs.com/SuzyCohen* or you can ask your doctor to become a practitioner of Rhein Labs and get a similar test for you. The key is to optimize testosterone to help reduce the antibody attack on your thyroid. This explain in part, why most men don't

Hashimoto's very often. In women who have low testosterone, the antibodies climb, especially if you ingest food antigens or have an infection. Too much testosterone will give you big zits on your face.

Vitamin D3. This nutrient balances an overactive immune system, so it can work in any autoimmune disease. It helps specifically by improving the number of T regulatory cells we have, which then go on to grow into various other cells that we need for a balanced immune system. (Doctors, this balances a Th1 or Th2 dominant condition, it's a modulator). Vitamin D is partially absorbed and assimilated in the small intestine and if you have any gut issues, this is compromised. If you're overweight, your fat cells will take up a lot of vitamin D and your need increases. The mere fact of aging, as well as taking antacids and fat blocking diet aids are 'drug muggers' of vitamin D, thus reducing absorption. Statins are also drug muggers of vitamin D so if you take one of those drugs to reduce cholesterol, you will automatically have less D in your body (and less CoQ10 too). If you have Hashi's (whether you know it or not) vitamin D will go a long way to put out the fire on your thyroid gland. It's hard to get too much D, usually we have too little. Read Chapter 5, *The Best Lab Tests,* to learn about the appropriate way to test for vitamin D. It's best evaluated with a ratio, not as a single number.

L.Glutamine. An inflamed or leaky gut will make every condition you have worse, and cause autoimmune diseases so you need to heal the gut. Glutamine is an amino acid that is essential for your gut lining. It helps keep the hairlike villi on the surface of your intestines very clean. It's like a vacuum for the shag rug in your gut. It reduces intestinal permeability and prevents too many of those undigested food particles from entering your blood stream. Excellent! Earlier in this chapter, I mentioned that the #1 thing you can do to help Hashi's is to avoid the food antigens, and right after that you need to heal your intestines to calm down the attack. It's like a weed. You can keep cutting the weed, but until you pull it out by the roots the problem doesn't stop. Healing the gut is the equivalent of pulling out the roots. You also need it to help generate glutathione which I talked about a minute ago (under selenium section). In some people with GAD snps (mutations), the glutamine can backfire and cause anxiety, irritability, insomnia, attention problems and even heaven-forbid seizures. You would know right off (within a few days) because you would feel bad after taking it; this is kind of rare but I want you to be aware that glutamine can have this effect on individuals who have genetic personalities which prevent them from breaking this down to GABA (a calming chemical) which is what most people do.

Probiotics. It's not normal to have a bowel movement every 3 days, it should be at least once daily or you are probably constipated. When constipated you hold on to toxins. Your health could improve dramatically if you take high quality probiotics that fertilize your garden of gut bacteria. Certain common strains improve the way your immune cells are made. Probiotics improve the amount of T4 to T3 conversion you get by about 20% so you might have more energy as a result. Probiotics improve regularity, and reduce symptoms of irritable bowel. They are critical to you if you have had your appendix removed (which is a warehouse to store beneficial bacteria). The beneficial flora in your intestinal tract have the ability to turn on and off the genes so you are not stuck with the genes (mutations) you were born with. Probiotics turn on healthy genes and reduce risk of other medical problems. They are absolutely fundamental to good health, and the first supplement I take in the morning. I always suggest you treat autoimmune disorders by starting in the gut. High quality probiotics are extremely important in telling your genes how to interact with the environment. You can read more about zonulin in Chapter 5, *The Best Lab Tests*. The brand I recommend (and represent) is Dr. Ohhira's Probiotic because I find that they support everyone's intestinal flora, they do not contain additives and they are guaranteed to be alive when you swallow them.

Digestive Enzymes. Your body has a digestive enzyme for gluten and casein (proteins from wheat and dairy) called "dipeptidyl peptidase-IV" or DPPIV. Yes, you actually make that but some of you are deficient. If those proteins are leaking out of your gut every time you eat a sandwich, then taking DPPIV can be impressively helpful. Remember, partially digested foods inflame you and attack your thyroid gland. You can take supplements that contain "DPPIV" and think of this digestive enzyme like PacMan chomping away on gluten and dairy. It's not an invitation to eat pizza but if you choose to, at least you know about this digestive enzyme. It's sold as Gluten-Ease by Enzymedica, and I put some of it into a special supplement which I formulated for people struggling with thyroid disease. It's called ThyroScript. *www.ScriptEssentials.com.*

Supplements to Avoid

You may want to avoid the following if you have Hashimoto's because they crank up a part of your immune system that you really need to calm down. Scientifically, this is explained as increasing Th1 dominance (and you want to calm it down). I would avoid or minimize the use of these herbs if you have a Th1 dominant (autoimmune) disease:

Alfalfa
Ashwagandha
Atragalus
Beta Glucan
Echinacea

Goldenseal
Licorice root (glycyrrhiza)
Lemon balm (Melissa officinalis)
Maitake mushroom

Supplements to Consider

You may want to try these if you have Hashimoto's because they improve functioning of a part of your immune system that you want to raise. Scientifically, this is explained as increasing Th2 dominance (and you want more of that). If you have an autoimmune disease, I would ask your doctor if it's okay to try any of these. Don't do it on your own because some autoimmune diseases fluctuate from Th1 to Th2 dominance, so this is just an idea (I don't know if it's right for you):

Curcumin
Grape seed extract
Green tea
Pycnogenol (pine bark)
Quercetin
Resveratrol
White willow bark

The Safest Supplements

Compounds that modulate the immune system, rather than speed it (or slow it) are to be thought of as 'big picture' supplements. The following should be fine whether or not you are Th1 or Th2 dominant because they are anti-inflammatory and they balance the see saw. Think of the following as immunomodulatory, which is different than immunostimulatory.

Probiotics
Vitamin D

Vitamin A
Vitamin E
Colostrum
Boswellia
Pancreatic Enzymes
Turmeric (and it's extract curcumin)
Essential Fatty Acids

What Else Can You Personally Do?

✓ Get a second or third opinion because each physician has a different toolbox.
✓ Get a copy of your own test results, so you can share, or do your own research.

Get tested properly. This can be a challenge because some physicians are unwilling to run specialized tests or they don't see the value in them as we do. You can buy some labs directly from trusted Internet sites that specialize in selling tests direct-to-consumer, here's my page: *www.DirectLabs.com/SuzyCohen.* I have set this up to help you get things done quickly, on your own time line. There are other direct-to-consumer lab sites too.

Ask for a trial course of medication even if your TSH, T3 or T4 lab values appear normal or high. Remember, as your antibodies are killing off the thyroid gland over time, you are dumping some of the thyroid hormone into your serum, so this means your labs will cause you to show higher T4 or T3 on the test. Medication might make you feel better.

Uncover chronic infections, sometimes that is what stimulates the auto-antibodies you see in Hashimoto's and Grave's disease. The best test for Lyme is through Igenex Labs in California. With a recent tick bite or sexual exposure, you can test with "iSpot Lyme" through Neuroscience.

Chapter 17

Graves' Disease

If your thyroid is overactive, it makes more thyroid hormone than your body needs. This condition is called hyperthyroidism. Excessive thyroid hormone can cause rapid unwanted weight loss, a fast heart rate, anxiety and irritability, sleep problems, shakiness, diarrhea, and feeling constantly hot or sweaty. Long term hyperthyroidism is associated with congestive heart failure or osteoporosis.

In this situation your thyroid gland produces too much thyroid hormone increasing all of your body's metabolic processes. Imagine everything on overdrive. A person with hypothyroidism can experience this condition by taking too much thyroid medicine, so be mindful of your dosage, and if you develop symptoms of hyperthyroidism, stop or back off.

Graves' disease is an autoimmune disorder where you make excessive thyroid hormone. Hashimoto's is an autoimmune disorder where you make too little thyroid hormone. You would think these two autoimmune disorders are opposites of each other, and to some extent they are because treatment approaches differ. To me, however, these conditions should be thought of as similar in one sense, because something you have been exposed to, or something you are eating is upsetting your immune system launching an attack your thyroid gland. The symptoms associated with high levels of thyroid hormone, termed "hyperthyroidism" are listed in

Table 10 Symptoms of Excessive Thyroid. These symptoms can occur if your medication dose is too high, or if you have Graves' disease.

Table 10. Symptoms of Excessive Thyroid

Anxiety
Double vision
Eyeballs that stick out (exophthalmos)
Diarrhea or frequent bowel movements
Big appetite
Hot or sweating all the time
Insomnia
Goiter (swollen neck because of an enlarged thyroid gland)
Irregular menstrual cycles
Nervousness
Shortness of breath
Tremor
Weight loss
Rapid or irregular heartbeat
Weakness or fatigue

Treatment of Graves' Disease

Your doctor will do a physical exam and may find that you have an increased heart rate. An exam of your neck, or an ultrasound may show that your thyroid gland is enlarged and makes your neck or throat swell (forming what's called a goiter). The standard treatment is to order blood tests such as TSH, T3 Free T4, TPO and Anti-TSH receptor antibodies, and others. Treatment is aimed at controlling the amount of thyroid hormone secreted, so you may get procedures or medications to reduce thyroxine (T4) secretion. Some people prefer natural protocols and others prefer a combination. For Grave's disease, your doctor may suggest other treatments to help you such radioactive iodine, antithyroid medicine or surgery. These carry risks. Even if they take out your thyroid gland I'd still be worried because your body is still host to the exposed toxin (or food antigen) that is causing the overactive immune system. So if you have a thyroidectomy, you will probably develop another autoimmune disease down the road. The key is to extinguish the fire, read Chapter 3. The best advice I can give you if you have Graves' is to eat an anti-inflammatory diet, make it as clean as possible.

If you have hyperthyroidism or Graves' disease, one simple thing to try is L-carnitine, a natural amino acid which interferes with T3's ability to transport into the cell. This supplement is generally well tolerated and safe. It has an added benefit of supporting heart and cholesterol health.

Thyroid Healthy Tip

Have you had surgery recently?

I often hear a person describe their symptoms of thyroid illness shortly after surgery, like weeks to months later. This is termed non-thyroidal illness and it happens after surgery. It's detrimental to NOT treat your condition. Your cells are hypothyroid and you are absolutely thyroid sick.

Dangers of Fluoride

Did you know that fluoride is one of the strongest ways to reduce thyroid hormone secretion? Fluoride was used as a drug to treat Graves' disease because it mimics the actions of TSH and when your body sees a lot of TSH, thyroid hormone production stops. So if fluoride is an impostor, posing as TSH, your body reacts the same. Fluoride is a halogen related compound just like iodine so if fluoride is present, your thyroid gland cannot make thyroid hormone anymore because the fluoride occupies the same spot that the iodine does. It knocks off the iodine halting thyroxine (T4) production. So having fluoride around is a double whammy, it acts like TSH and it competes for iodine. Two strikes. The third strike is that fluoride deposits itself in your pineal gland and reduces your production of melatonin. You need that hormone for deep sleep. Isn't your sleep bad enough with your thyroid situation? You can understand now why I ask you to avoid fluoride dental products, tap water that is fluoridated and all fluorinated drugs. You should avoid them if you're healthy, but especially if you have Hashimoto's or hypothyroidism. See page 97 for Fluorinated drugs. This is why iodine can help offset damage done by halides. The United States Recommended Daily Intake is 150 µg iodine per day and this falls way short of what you need to protect yourself form iodine deficiency. This amount may be good to keep you from developing a deficiency, but it does nothing to promote health. Dosage is very individual, it could be anything from 500 µg up to 12.5 mg per day! I know that is a huge dosage range, but that's because it is based upon your individual lab tests.

Parathyroid Disease

This is another set of glands that reside against your thyroid gland and they produce hormones that control the amount of calcium found in your blood and your bones. The name is confusing, but the parathyroid glands do not affect thyroid hormone, at least not a whole lot. There has been some research done lately and it appears that goiters, Graves' disease and Hashimoto's disease (Chapter 17) are associated with hyperparathyroidism (overactive parathyroid gland). It's not always the case, however an association has been found in elderly women.

I don't want to spend a whole lot of time on the parathyroid gland, I only mention it here because surgery or radiation treatments for thyroid cancer and Graves' disease may harm your parathyroid gland. Then, it becomes the collateral damage from these thyroid treatments. So nourishing your thyroid gland, and doing everything you can to keep it healthy protects your parathyroid gland as well. If you have high calcium in your bloodstream, it could be a parathyroid problem. Your parathyroid glands may malfunction and cause vague symptoms that could be attributed to tons of other conditions. Nevertheless, I want you to know what some of those symptoms are for further evaluation. The tests they use to check for parathyroid illness are blood tests, and pretty straight-forward.

Symptoms of Parathyroid Illness

Anxiety
Back pain
Cracked teeth
Fatigue
Gastric reflux disease
Hostility
Insomnia
Headaches
Heart palpitations
High blood pressure
Muscle pain
Obsessive or compulsive behavior
Osteopenia, osteoporosis

PTU for Graves' Disease

With hypothyroidism, it's hard to convince some doctors to test you. If they realized that rT3 is a thyroid blocker, and that it's your anti-thyroid hormone, testing for rT3 would be offered more frequently as part of your total work up. I'm telling you rT3 is a more potent blocker of T4 to T3 conversion than PTU (propylthiouracil), the very drug used to treat high thyroid in Graves' disease! I'm saying that rT3 suppresses levels of thyroid hormone so well that it's better than a drug! If that's the case why isn't this biomarker routinely measured for people with hypothyroidism in every doctor's office in America? Read about the benefits of measuring rT3 in Chapter 5, *The Best Lab Tests*. Know that you make this rT3 whenever you are stressed (high cortisol), or when you become mineral deficient. You make this rT3 when you take certain T4 drugs. As for PTU? My warning to you is to be careful if you have to take it and get routine liver function tests every 3 months. In 2009 the FDA issued a warning about liver failure and death.

Methimazole & Carbamazole and Graves' Disease

Carbamazole and methimazole are prescription drugs used to treat Graves' disease. They are referred to as antithyriod drugs. The Carbamazole is a prodrug, it is taken by mouth and after your body absorbs it, it's converted in the body to methimazole. So methimazole (which is a drug all by itself) is really doing the work, and it suppresses your natural production of thyroid hormone from your gland, and also conversion in the tissues. The caution with these drugs is that they are "azole" drugs and some people are allergic to azole drugs. These should not be used in pregnancy as a general rule. Sometimes you hear of sudden blood-related side effects like agranulocytosis or neutropenia which can occur at any time of treatment. These are both names for a condition that is severe and it reduces certain white blood cells in the body.

Children and Graves' Disease

Children will often get bulging eyes, a condition termed "orbitopa-thy" and it's embarrassing for them. Adults get this too, and it's commonly associated with Graves' disease. You can imagine the upper eyelid being retracted back, with the bulging eyeballs, swelling and conjunctivitis. German researchers conducted a very interesting clinical trial. This study included 422 serum samples from 157 children with Grave's Disease, 101control participants with other thyroid and non-thyroid autoimmune diseases, and

50 healthy children. The researchers measured various markers of thyroid function including Thyroid Stimulating antibodies or TSAb in the blood. Almost all of the kids (94%) with Grave's related eye disease had a much more serious autoimmune attack going on than the children with Graves' disease that did not affect the eye. When the kids were treated, they showed almost 70% reduction in those antibodies (TSAb) so treatment can really make a difference if your child has eye protrusion. It probably works the same for adults!

Thyroid Healthy Tip

Feeling anxious from hyperthyroidism, Graves' disease or too much thyroid medicine today? Theanine may help. It's a natural remedy sold as a dietary supplement, and it occurs naturally in green tea.

Bugleweed for Graves' Disease

Bugleweed also known as Gypsy Weed is your antithyroid herb, so it's helpful if you take too much thyroid medicine, or if you have Graves' disease. I love this herb if you want something natural to reduce T4 production, but of course ask a holistic-minded physician about all changes to your protocol. Bugleweed is fabulous for premenstrual syndrome (PMS), heavy bleeding during your period, breast pain and insomnia. Taking too much bugleweed can enlarge your thyroid gland so be careful, dosage adjustments are key to making this work. It is available in many supplement forms including a pure liquid herbal extract by Herb Pharm which I like because it is not fumigated or irradiated. It comes as a liquid dropper and you put some drops in a little water and drink it several times a day. Bugleweed can help manage the symptoms of hyperthyroidism, especially palpitations, and you don't necessarily need it forever if you are addressing the lifestyle factors that actually fix the autoimmune attack. For instance, if you fix that leaky gut and cut out foods that spark you, the antibodies go down and you need less and less Bugleweed (or PTU, or methimazole). I'm saying that as you heal, you should become less dependent on herbal medications or prescribed ones. Of course, your physician will work with you on weaning off. It's not an abrupt thing. One more caution, Bugleweed is contraindicated in pregnant and nursing women. It's less potent than a drug, so, side effects are not as common with the herb. It all comes down to risk versus benefits of each.

Motherwort for Graves' Disease

Motherwort (Leonurus cardiaca) is a natural herb that can help you if you if you have Graves' disease. It spreads calm and joy throughout your body. It helps with heart rate because it is kind of like a natural beta blocker (like propranolol, the drug). It can help with tremors. Imagine this herb as a general heart and mind tonic. It's less potent than the antithyroid drugs like PTU or methimazole, so, this means it has fewer if any dangerous side effects common to medications. You can take Motherwort with Bugleweed if you need to, so long as your doctor approves of what you are doing. It's not for me to decide. This is contraindicated in pregnancy, however some doctors allow it while nursing. This is up to your holistic doctor to decide.

Sunshine Vitamin for Graves' Disease

We know that vitamin D deficiency is associated with many autoimmune diseases like rheumatoid arthritis, systemic lupus erythematosus (lupus), inflammatory bowel disease, multiple sclerosis, Hashimoto's thyroiditis and Type 1 diabetes. What about Graves' disease?

Researchers evaluated 26 female patients with newly diagnosed Graves' disease and 46 healthy females (considered the controls because they had normal thyroid function). The data collected proved that women with Graves' Disease had significantly lower vitamin D levels compared to the control group. In fact, 65.4% of the Graves' disease patients were considered vitamin D deficient compared to only 32.4% of the control participants. The deficiency even affected the size of the thyroid gland, causing it to swell bigger in the patients with the lowest amount of D. Vitamin D is powerful and supports the immune system, especially in autoimmune thyroid illness. It specifically seems to control the inflammatory response in thyroid cells and T helper cells by reducing the production of pain-causing chemicals (called cytokines). I think this study really defines vitamin D's role as immunoprotective and anti-inflammatory. I suspect that deficiencies contribute to the onset of autoimmune diseases including Graves' disease. Maybe it's preventable if you keep your D levels up, it's worth a try. Check your levels, you might feel better with a serum level of 50 or above. To get that you may need to supplement with a high-quality vitamin D. Please read about *how to test for vitamin D properly in Chapter 5, The Best Lab Tests.*

More Natural Remedies

Options, I love them. For that reason I'm going to just point out some other natural remedies which could help, but please research these on your own. All but one of these are sold at health food stores nationwide. Ask a practitioner if it's okay for you with your current situation and allergy history:

- ✓ Digestive Enzymes to reduce inflammation and calm the autoimmune attack
- ✓ Bromelain to reduce pain and inflammation
- ✓ Lemonbalm tea
- ✓ Passionflower herb
- ✓ L-carnitine
- ✓ Low dose naltrexone, a medication to calm the immune system (page 152)

Part V
Thyroid Treatment

Chapter 18

Medications

Many of you feel better once you start medication. We are calling them medications but for all practical purposes these could be thought of as "hormone replacement."

Many factors contribute to your recovery, and depend on the type of medication you take. Your doctor will determine which medication you need, and the appropriate dose. You'll continue to see your doctor to make dosage adjustments, especially in the beginning. If you have any big life changes, your dosage may need tune ups. We are all unique with individual sensitivities to the amount of T4, T3 and even the fillers (inactive ingredients) in the pills.

We all react differently to the same medications. The dosages that are ideal for each of us will also vary. Our individual differences, and our specialness is what makes finding the right thyroid hormone replacement medication very tricky. Get it right and you feel amazing, get it wrong and you feel lousy. If you take the wrong dose, it could harm you! Soon, you will read about the different types of medications.

Can You Lose Weight on Thyroid?

I'm often asked if taking high dosages of thyroid medication can help you lose weight. The question is pondered right before you want to attend your 20 year high school reunion or a wedding where you want to squeeze into a dress that doesn't fit you anymore. I hear ya! But the answer is no, you need to stick to the dosage that was prescribed for you. Doubling up or taking excessive dosages in an effort to lose weight quickly can cause insomnia, agitation and heart arrhythmias. It is not good for you, it is very dangerous and can land you in the hospital. Thyroid hormone has widespread effects from head to toe and you should not take dosages, or pills that were not prescribed for you.

We Are All Unique

Our uniqueness is what prevents me from giving you a clear plan of action. I know you as a reader want a simple plan of action like "Take this drug, at this dose and all your symptoms will go away!" I can't do that because what works for you, doesn't work for your best friend. Some of you want me to say, "Such-and-such drug is the absolute best drug on the market!" No such thing because "best" is a relative term, what's best for you is not best for the next person. We are individuals. Think of your fingerprint. No two are the same. That is the case with your body. Personalized medicine is the wave of the future. Even the American business-man and entrepreneur, Mark Cuban from Shark Tank, openly says that personalized medicine is the "next big thing."

You have a fingerprint of hormones, and function of liver, kidneys and GI tract. You have a fingerprint of beneficial bacteria (probiotics), you have so many unique factors, there is no way to offer one plan to millions of you reading my book, all over the world. What I can tell you is to follow my "Script" plan in Chapter 24. Go slowly when trying new medications and be gentle with yourself. You'll have to experiment with the medications and supplements and there's a trend over time, don't make a judgment after 1 day of a particular medicine. Keep a diary if you can. It's taken you years to get to this point, and it can't be fixed overnight, or with one magic thyroid pill. The first step to getting thyroid healthy is understanding what is going on and feeling empowered to do something about it.

Does Thyroid Medicine Even Work?

Yes it does, if you take the right one. The key is taking the right medicine for yourself. The studies show that little benefit is seen with thyroid replacement, because the researchers are using T4 in their studies and the results are not so great. That would be expected wouldn't it? Even you know this now because you have been reading my book, and learning that T4 is biologically inactive, it doesn't do anything until it's converted to T3. So if you replace active T3 hormone in a person, with a do-nothing hormone (T4), what would you expect the result to be? Right! Nothing. It's like replacing the gas in your car with windshield wiper fluid, and complaining the car doesn't work. It's not going to work until your car figures out a way to convert that windshield wiper fluid into gasoline so the car can run! Now, let's put gas in your gas tank (instead of wiper fluid). What I'm trying to say is put T3 into people, rather than T4. What do you think happens now? Think about it, T3 is what you make, it is clinically bioavailable to you, no conversion necessary. It's going to work much better right?

This is so dang simple to understand that even my friend's daughter who is 12 years old understood it when I taught her. It took me 5 minutes to teach her, that's it! Why is thyroid replacement given in the form of T4 drugs forever and ever? It's okay for a while, or in combination with some T3.

Your level of T4 does not reflect what is happening in your body, in your tissues which is really what you need to know! Our "health care" is really messed up isn't it? As a result, you miss out on so many good things in life, or you push through. Thankfully you have my book to teach you how to test and interpret labs correctly, and how to choose medicine wisely. The old school thinking is preventing you from getting thyroid healthy.

This is why so many of you are sick and tired, and spending years in a virtual emotional coma, holding on to weight, crying, anxious, tossing and turning at night? Getting adequate hormone replacement medications can breathe life into you. I'm not just referring to thyroid, I also think you could benefit from bio-identical forms of other hormones like estrogen, progesterone, testosterone or DHEA. Natural adaptogens that support adrenal health is imperative. A good holistic-minded doctor can uncover abnormalities in all of these areas very easily, usually within a week or two if they know how to test.

Medication Basics

Depending on the type of medication prescribed, you may need to go to a regular pharmacy, or a specialized compounding pharmacy. Thyroid replacement is given by oral medication, not intravenously so it's very easy for you to take. If you have specific allergies to ingredients in pills such as lactose, gluten, or artificial dyes you'll probably want to get your medication compounded by a pharmacy that specializes in making 'clean' capsules that are free of common allergenic ingredients.

The longer that you have been thyroid sick or hypothyroid, the more likely you will need a combination of T4/T3 medication, or pure T3 for awhile, your worst choice would be pure T4 drugs because chronic illness causes slow conversion of T4 to T3.

You see, a healthy person should convert 50% of their T4 drug to active T3 to feel well, but if you have been ill for a long time, you can't do that well. For instance, and this is not all inclusive, but if you have a pain syndrome, chronic Lyme, fibromyalgia, chronic fatigue syndrome or autoimmune illness, you can't convert it effectively. If you have a lot of stress in your life, or you are a caregiver, or you travel a lot, the same applies. This is why T3 medication, or combinations of T4/T3 drugs work better for you.

Determine Your Dose on 5 Key Factors

1. Your age! Older folks need to start with lower doses
2. Conditions you have such as diarrhea, Celiac, cirrhosis and pregnancy
3. History of heart problems because that warrants a lower dose, and slower titration up
4. Other medications you take
5. Severity of your symptoms

7 Rules When Taking Medication

Rule #1 If your dose is once daily, then take it first thing, upon arising, on an empty stomach. Do not brush your teeth for a half an hour if possible (the fluoride may interfere). Drink only water.

Rule #2 If your dosage is twice daily, the first pill is taken upon arising, and the second pill is taken between noon and 3pm sometimes (unless your doctor advises different). Do not take your second pill too late in the day because it could interfere with sleep. With pure T3 drugs, you often see those prescribed throughout the day, and if it is not stimulating for you, then it is alright to take your second dose (or third dose) at bedtime. Talk to your doctor and ask how it is recommended for you. Note your reactions to it, and how well you can get to sleep. Refreshing, restorative sleep is imperative to your well-being.

Rule #3 Do not take multivitamins, especially those with minerals at the same time as your medicine. The minerals tie up the hormone and reduce absorption.

Rule #4 Do not take iron or calcium supplements within 2 hours of your thyroid medication. With this rule in mind, do not drink milk either, because of the calcium. It reduces absorption.

Rule #5 Do not drink coffee or caffeinated tea within 1 hour of your thyroid medication.

Rule #6 If you're resting pulse is very high, above 80 or 90, it is a sign your dosage is too high. You may need to back off your medicine or take Bugleweed for a day or two, see page 165 for more on that. Of course, you will need to alert your doctor about your experience and symptoms of hyperthyroidism.

Rule #7 If you decide to take a new supplement with your medication, and you've been stable for a long time, make sure you keep a diary or log each day. If you develop signs or symptoms of hyperthyroidism, it means that your supplement is helping you, and you need to back off the medicine. Naturally, this all occurs with your doctor's blessing and supervision.

Table 11. Food & Drug Interactions with Thyroid Medications

The following medications and foods may interfere with your medicine, specifically T4 absorption.

Antacids (Tums, Maalox)
Cholesterol binding drugs (Cholestyramine, Colestipol)
Iron supplements
Calcium-fortified foods like orange juice
Calcium supplements
H2 blockers (acid blockers like Zantac, Tagamet, Pepcid)
High fiber diet or Metamucil
Proton pump inhibitors (acid blockers like Nexium, Prilosec, Prevacid)
Seizure medications (phenobarbital, phenytoin, carbamazepine)
Soybean-derived foods (edemame, soy milk, tofu, tempeh)
Sucralfate (Carafate)

Let's Meet the Medications

T4 Medications

Examples: Levothyroxine, L thyroxine or thyroxine sodium
Synthroid, Levoxyl, Unithroid and Tirosint in the United
States.
Tirosint is a hypoallergenic gel cap that is believed to be
better absorbed.

Pure T4 drugs are sold all around the world by other names:

Berlthyrox, Droxine, Eferox, Elthyrone, Eltroxin, Eutirox,
Euthyrox, Letrox, Levaxin, Levotirox, Levothyrox,
Levotiroxina, Oroxine, T4KP, Thevier, Throxinique,
Thyradin, Thyradin S, Thyrax, Thyrax Duotab, Thyro-Tabs,
Thyro-4, Thyrosit, Thyroxine, Thyroxine-Natrium, Tiroidine

Discussion: Are T4 Medications Right For You?

Some people do fine and convert these T4 drugs to their active
T3 counterpart, especially in the beginning of treatment. The
healthier you are, the more likely these drugs will work well for
you. I personally do not recommend them if you've been ill for
more than 6 months. If you are "thyroid sick" (thyroid resistant)
you would not receive benefits from T4 medications because they
don't give you any T3.

A study published in *European Journal of Endocrinology*, a
highly respected and reputable endocrinology journal, found
that combination drugs such as T4/T3 is superior to T4 drugs
(Levothyroxine). If you're on a T4 medication and your rT3 comes
back high, that means your cells are hungry for T3. You could
very well add in a T3 medication (such as Cytomel) and take it
along with your T4 med (like Synthroid). Doing this allows you
to make easy adjustments to either your T4 drug or your T3 drug.
Why wouldn't you just switch to a T4/T3 combination and take
one pill? You certainly could, but I would do that only after you've

figured out how much T4 and T3 you need each day. This is unique to you. The dosage may change by the week, especially if you begin juicing, detoxifying your body of toxins, improving your diet and taking supplements. Once you settle upon a dose, you could get a combination T4/T3 medication at any compounding pharmacy if your doctor calls it in. Another simple option is to take natural desiccated thyroid pills which are available at commercial pharmacies.

Does Synthroid Go Into Your Cells?

Some of it can yes, but the problem is that if it does not go into the cell, you will convert some of it to rT3. You may convert a lot of it to rT3, and if you recall that is what I affectionately call your hibernation hormone because excessive amounts makes you tired and sleepy. It doesn't usually penetrate the cell very well unless you're transport system is in great shape, and it might be if you're feeling awesome. If you feel good on Synthroid, that means it's getting into your cell and I'd stay on it, but if you're feeling bad, you may need adrenal support and some pure T3. You may also benefit from a T4/T3 combination like natural desiccated thyroid (NDT). My rule of thumb: The worse you feel, the more T3 you need to balance the T4.

If Your T4 Is Low, Would Synthroid Help?

Who cares if your T4 is low, you only need that to convert to T3? You don't need to take T4 if your physiological levels are low. It's the Free T3 you have to concern yourself with because that is your active hormone. Most people have no trouble making T4 unless they have lost their thyroid gland, or they are iodine deficient. Taking iodine could help. And to directly answer this question, yes, if you need T4 in your body, Synthroid is a good choice.

Is Synthroid Bio-identical to Endogenous T4 in the Body?

Yes.

What Are the Inactive Ingredients of Synthroid?

Acacia, confectioner's sugar (contains corn starch), lactose, monohydrate, magnesium stearate, povidone, and talc. There are also various different artificial coloring agents depending on the strength.

T4/T3 Combination Drugs

These can be broken down into 2 subcategories, natural and synthetic. Natural thyroid medications are derived from the glands of animals (usually pigs). These types of medications are referred to as "Natural Desiccated Thyroid" or NDT medications.

Examples: Amour Thyroid by Forest Laboratories
Nature-Throid by RLC Labs
WP Thyroid (formerly Westhroid Pure) by RLC Labs
Thyrolar, a synthetic combination of T4 and T3 in a fixed
4:1 ratio
Compounded T4/T3 (made by compounding pharmacies,
ratio customized)
Compounded T4/T3 Long-Acting (made by compounding
pharmacies, ratio customized)

Discussion: Are T4/T3 Medications Right For You?

There can be significant differences between compounding pharmacies so if you switch pharmacies (because of coupons, or pricing, or because you've moved), there may be differences in how you feel. My suggestion is to stay with the pharmacy that creates the form you feel best on. My other suggestion is to stick with the fixed ratios if those work well for you. But are T4/T3 drugs right for you? T4/T3 medications act like natural "hormone replacement" for lack of a better word, these are combinations of two hormones you naturally make and need. The trouble with T4 drugs is poor conversion to T3 so these combo pills solve that.

Many of you may finally feel relief from symptoms if you switch from a pure T4 drug to a combination of T4 and T3 like Armour. This drug contains the combination of pork-derived T4 and T3 that your body recognizes because it's animal derived and similar to your own hormone. Insurance will cover medications like this when dispensed from a retail pharmacy, and sometimes even if you get the compounded version. Compounded T4/T3 combinations offer a great advantage for some of you because the ratio is customized.

Remember, these drugs come in a fixed ratio, you can't adjust yourself if you want to take more T3 or less T4. Because you can't bio-individualize it, there could be less satisfaction for some of you who require much higher doses of T3. For people who have conversion issues, you will have trouble converting the T4 in the tablet to T3, and then getting it into the cell. Your natural secretion of thyroid hormone occurs in a pulsed fashion, it's not secreted from your thyroid gland all day long. There are doctors and experts who are openly not in love with T4/T3 drugs because they perceive T4 as nothing more than a vehicle to get to T3. If you recall from the very beginning, I mentioned that T4 (thyroxine) hormone was necessary to activate riboflavin to another form called "flavin adenine dinucleotide" or FAD. I wish you could buy FAD but you cannot. You have to create that inside your body. You need T4 to create it, not T3, and so I don't want you to walk away from my book, or from a physician thinking T4 is useless or worthless. It is meaningful to people with methylation defects and there are millions of you with that genetic problem, and you don't even know. You can take a blood test to find out. If you are thyroid sick, and you have a methylation defect, you really need adequate physiological levels of Free T4 to make this special ribo-flavin vitamin, which in turn 'takes out the garbage' of your cells. It detoxifies the cells in your body. I personally supplement with the active supplemental form called riboflavin 5' phosphate because I have a methylation snp (mutation) and want to maintain my thyroid levels.

Nature-Throid and Armour Thyroid are 2 different drugs made by two different companies. They are both porcine (pig) derived so on occasion you hear of someone being allergic to that or to a filler. Your mitochondria are little motors in your cell, you have 3 and a half pounds of motors, and you need them to run well or you are tired. Perhaps this is an unspoken benefit of NDT drugs that we will one day hear more about. You heard it here first. Desiccated thyroid drugs are made according to quality controlled standards contrary to what some people say. Taking Selenium with your medication improves T3 conversion.

Are People Allergic To NDT Drugs?

Yes, some are due to the fact that it's a pig-derived glandular extract, and it's not bio-identical. Natural desiccated thyroid or NDT is one of the oldest drugs known to medicine. Some people are allergic to pork and don't realize that and they take these desiccated drugs and itch all over. It's not just pork allergies, you can become allergic to any medication, porcine-derived or not. The reaction could be anything from an annoying itch, to a full body rash, swollen lips, hives, all the way to life-threatening anaphylaxis with any medication. NDT drugs contain four naturally occurring forms of thyroid hormone, T1, T2, T3 and T4. We usually only talk about the T3 and T4 in these drugs though, you rarely hear T1 or T2 mentioned. There are studies to show that your T2 hormone activates your mitochondria, but this is very new science and you don't usually hear about it.

But it's not just the glandular drugs that cause reactions in the sensitive, it's also synthetic drugs. Most all prescription thyroid medications contain cornstarch, lactose and gluten which you may be reacting to. Most hypothyroid patients have sensitivities to gluten, which will make you sensitive to corn, dairy (casein and lactose), and other grains. The most hypoallergenic one is "WP Thyroid" made by RLC Labs, because it contains only 2 inactive ingredients, both natural (inulin from chicory root, and medium chain triglycerides from coconut). It comes in 8 different strengths making dose titration very simple. Armour Thyroid has dealt with the most backlash in terms of fillers. So much so, that in 2008, the manufacturers of Armour reformulated their product, reducing the amount of dextrose while increasing the methylcellulose in the filler. The reports flooded in, and people said the new formula was either fantastic or horrible, depending on which component of the pill they were sensitive too.

Why Isn't My NDT Drug Working Anymore?

It's a great question. I can shed light on that. First, read through the following comments and see which you identify with:

I feel worse on thyroid medicine.

NDT does nothing for me, I feel the same.

NDT (or T3 drugs) make me irritable, anxious or give me tremors.

My heart rate (or resting pulse) is very high on my thyroid medicine.

I experienced a panic attack!

I feel nauseous on NDT or other thyroid medicine.

I get more headaches on thyroid medicine.

The reason for the failure of NDT thyroid medication could be very correctible if you know what to look for. You may have poor adrenal function. This is a big one, I cannot emphasize it enough. When you're stressed, your thyroid medicine doesn't work. You may notice no benefit from your thyroid medicine because it's not going into the cell to help you. That's what happens if you are iron deficient. So if you take NDT, you may notice it causing shakiness, irritability, headaches, insomnia and heart beat irregularities which could mean you're iron deficient and/or the dose is too high. (This exact situation can occur with Levothyroxine too). Some people take NDT and feel jittery or shaky within a few hours but then it stops. This is often related to the T3 burning off. Remember, NDT medications are a combination of T4 and T3, and the T3 goes into your bloodstream immediately so you can get the jittery effect. As it gets metabolized (burns off), you are left with the T4 portion which is converted slowly. In this case, you may want to lower your NDT dose, or switch from NDT to a long-acting version of T3, or go back to pure T4 drugs.

If you have low stomach acid (hypochlorhydria), you absorb less medication and fewer minerals from your food which you need to make thyroid hormone. This translates to chronic fatigue. So be careful not to blame medications, as in "These drugs don't work for me!" when it's really about you, and your adrenals, your intestinal health and nutrient depletions. Get those in order and then your thyroid replacement medications will suddenly work better. Your doctor has to do the conversion for you, as a general rule, 25 mcg of pure T3 is about equal to 1 grain of NDT, and 1 grain of NDT equals about 65 mg. 1 grain of most NDT drugs contain 38 mcg of T4 and 9 mcg of T3. Switching from NDT to T3 requires practitioner supervision. I've seen many doctors suggest that you reduce your NDT dose by half. Take that for 1 week, then begin 10 mcg of T3 (with your NDT). Reduce NDT dosage and simultaneously add more T3 each week until you take about 25 mcg of T3 to replace every 1 grain NDT that is dropped. Monitor morning body temperature and symptoms. T3 medications can be split up during the day if needed.

Pure T3 Drugs

Examples: Cytomel (brand of liothyronine)
Liothyronine
Compounded T3 by any compounding pharmacy
Compounded long-acting (LA) T3 by any compounding
    pharmacy

Discussion: Are T4/T3 Medications Right For You?

Taking T3 medicines give you the advantage of not worrying whether or not you can convert T4 to T3, because you are taking T3 directly. I like this option for those of you that are thyroid sick. It could help you, and it's not that you need a T3 drug long-term, I don't think that's good, but for a little while, perhaps 2 to 6 months to restore physiological levels. Routine evaluations of your Free T3 will be needed.

Cytomel from the pharmacy is short-acting so you need to take it several times a day but this can cause heart problems, if your dose isn't steady all day long. A stable body level of T3 will reduce these heart-related side effects. Time release (termed "LA") is available from a compounding pharmacy, but sometimes the pharmacies put too much of the long-acting compound in it and then it doesn't work well. The long-acting compound is called Methocel™ and causes drug release slowly over time. In our case, the drug is T3 hormone. The Methocel™ binds up some of the T3 in the pill so you absorb less. It's not a major problem but I want you to know about that in case you are switching over from a time release (long acting) form ofT3 to another type of medication. Other ways to reduce thyroid medication absorption include having Celiac, malabsorption, gastric bypass, intestinal permeability, bacterial or yeast overgrowth in the gut, low digestive enzymes and pancreatitis.

Cytomel contains "liothyronine sodium" also called LT3, and this is a synthetic form of a natural thyroid hormone. It's short-acting. Temporary hair loss has been reported. Cytomel can be taken alone or added to T4 drugs like Synthroid. Cytomel is a conventional standard drug you get from the pharmacy, and compounded T3 dosages are created by hand based upon your specific dose. They are not exactly interchangeable because the Compounded T3 is less potent than Cytomel. Cytomel, contains modified food starch, which could mean it has gluten or corn. Switching from T3 drugs to NDT drugs can be challenging, so your doctor has to do the conversion for you. As a general rule, 25 mcg of pure T3 is about equal to 1 grain of NDT, and 1 grain of NDT equals about 65 mg. It depends on the specific drug.

Thyroid Healthy Tip

Be super careful with your medication and avoid taking high doses. Don't leave it near the children either. Thyrotoxicosis factitia known more commonly as a "Thyroid Storm" is a dangerous condition that results from taking too much medication and spiking your thyroid levels rapidly. It's basically an overdose! The symptoms to look out for include anxiety, nervousness, palpitations, hand tremor, staring off into space and other signs of hyperthyroidism. The risk of heart attack is extremely high. It's a trip to the hospital. Emergency room doctors often administer high-dose iodine which shuts down the thyroid.

Should You Take Medications The Morning of Your Blood Test?

Do you take Synthroid or pure T4 drugs? Then it doesn't matter if you skip your T4 medicine or not. You could take that and still take your blood test without worrying about the results.

Do you take Cytomel or Compounded T3? This means you need to skip your medication the morning of your test, and take it after your blood test.

Do you take Natural Desiccated Thyroid (Armour, Nature-Throid)? Then it's okay to take your medication, but only if you're taking the blood test right away. If you're going to be longer than 3 or 4 hours after taking your medicine, take it later.

This Is One Drug You Should Never Take

Do you have poor immunity, or get sick frequently? Have you ever had sinusitis, an earache, or a bladder or urinary tract infection? How about a kidney infection? Some antibiotics worry me, in particular the fluoroquinolones or "quinolones" for short. This is a category of prescription antibiotics that I recommend as your last resort. The quinolone antibiotics are built with a fluoride backbone, which helps them penetrate tissues that other antibiotics can't get into such as your urinary tract, your brain, kidney, prostate, and your thyroid. They were intended to be used for life-threatening infections because they get into every single cell in your body, nothing escapes them. Some of you don't even know you got the drug because it was given to you in the hospital as part of your pre-op or during surgery! Find out if you took it. Even though the drugs were originally intended for life-threatening infections, today they are practically given out like candy from a Pez dispenser, for mild infections that other antibiotics could help. What's the big deal?

For one thing, combining quinolone antibiotics with Levothyroxine (a T4 drug) may lead to reduced absorption of thyroid medicine and cause changes in TSH. Further, fluoride is extremely poisonous to your thyroid. Because of the fluoride backbone, I worry about it harming your thyroid gland. I don't like fluoride, or fluorine, or anything related to fluoride coming anywhere near your thyroid gland, period! Fluoride damages the pineal gland too.

These issues are the least of my worries! Use of potent antibiotics to treat a minor infection could cause life-long, scary neurological, abdominal and mental disturbances. Some children and adults have taken a course of these antibiotics and reported life-long problems, sudden severe insomnia, hypnic jerks, tendon and cartilage tears, brain fog, weird sensations like bugs crawling on you, headaches, buzzing, pain, tinnitus (ear ringing), face-down fatigue, moving abdominal pain and every thyroid symptom possible. The difficulty is that your MRIs and blood work will all be pretty much normal. The drugs are called antibiotics but they work similar to chemotherapy, breaking apart DNA strands by affecting the enzyme DNA gyrase.

You would never connect this nasty array of symptoms to your antibiotic. Because the symptoms are occasionally delayed, occurring after you're done with the antibiotic. Go to my website, *SuzyCohen.com* and read the article entitled "Fluoroquinolones: Some Medications Scare Me." This article could change your life. Perhaps you got "floxed", that is the term used by floxies who got hurt from these antibiotics. Refer to Table 12 Fluoroquinolone or "Quinolone" Antibiotics, to see if you've ever taken one of these drugs, even just one pill. Four medications have been yanked off the market, and the remaining drugs have a "Black Box" warning on them from the FDA. The quinolone drugs are known by many other brand names around the world. They are commonly used in children (Egad! That scares me!) for simple earaches and eye infections. You'll see "otic" on the label for ear drops and "oph- thalmic" for the eye drops. I know some of you moms stash medicine for your child, "just in case" the infection comes back. Ask your pharmacist if the medicine you have is a fluoroquinolone or look it up online. Better yet, ask your pediatrician for an alternative. Just so you know, the "Cortisporin" brand of drops is not a fluoroquinolone, so I feel good about those.

Table 12. Fluoroquinolone or "Quinolone" Antibiotics

Ciprofloxacin	Cipro, Ciloxan eye drops
Levofloxacin	Levaquin, Quixin
Moxifloxacin	Avelox, Vigamox eye drops
Norfloxacin	Noroxin
Ofloxacin	Ocuflox, Floxin, Floxin Otic, Floxacin
Trovafloxacin	Trovan
alatrofloxacin	Trovan IV

What Did I Personally Do?

You may be wondering what I ultimately took myself to optimize my thyroid. It was a pure T3 medication compounded by a pharmacy, at 5 mcg each morning. I also took high doses of vitamin C, and natural adrenal adaptogens, and I switched those around a lot, every 2 months. I like ashwagandha the most, but also tried a month on rhodiola, a month on Panax ginseng, then licorice and schizandra herb. And I rotated because some of them gave me pimples. Each of these has their own incredible health benefits, so you should research them and ask your practitioner which one (or which combination) would suit you best. I found 10 minutes each day to break away from work and just go breathe or meditate. I avoided exercising for awhile because I didn't want to push my body too hard. I slowly eased back into exercise. I started with yoga, and then got back into dance. Today, I feel really pretty good. I ate gluten free for a couple of years, and then switched to Paleo for another 2 years. I began juicing and eating more organic foods so it wasn't all meat, but when I did eat meat it was clean. And I made a concerted effort to watch funny programs on TV, instead of the news so that I could keep my spirit up. The body wants to heal itself, it tries very hard, we just have to get out of its way by giving it the foundation to repair itself instead of more and more chemicals.

Chapter 19

Supplements to Feel Thyroid Healthy

I'm a big advocate of supplements for thyroid support, and some do have merit. Most supplements don't really *make use* of the thyroid hormone you naturally produce, they give you cofactors to help you make more thyroid, as in T4. You'll see supplements everywhere that promote production of T4 and by now, you know that thyroid illness is related to inflammation, food allergens (like gluten or casein) and the inability to get your T3 into your cell which turn the lights and power on. Remember my example of the house being locked? If not, read Chapter 3, *Thyroid on Fire*.

Probiotics Influence Thyroid Levels

Probiotics can make a big difference because 20% of your inactive T4 is converted to active T3 in your gut. Probiotics help you activate your thyroid hormone. Sometimes this is all a person needs to normalize a mild deficiency that is why I'm starting this chapter with probiotics. It would be lovely if we all had enough beneficial flora, but unfortunately, we are all woefully inadequate when it comes to good gut bugs.

I love this simple fix because probiotics are incredible immune boosters and they help you utilize the thyroid hormone you make, rather than letting it go to waste.

As you've learned, I am a firm believer that you need to make your thyroid hormone work for you, rather than keep pumping in more and more. Probiotics do just that, they help you activate thyroid hormone that would otherwise go to waste. You should take a high-quality probiotic because, after all, these are bacteria; you only want to take bacteria that is common to your gastro-intestinal flora. You don't want to dump a bazillion germs in, that are perceived as foreign strains. The goal with probiotic supplementation should be to make your own garden of bacteria flourish, not drop in a bunch of weeds. I get irritated with brands that have all sorts of weird strains. Your body needs to recognize the strains or there could be some backlash, for instance, a low grade autoimmune assault because your body is trying to figure out why some weird-looking bacteria is in you all of a sudden.

Did you know that all medicines are drug muggers of intestinal flora? In Chapter 7 of my Drug Muggers book, I have a complete discussion of probiotics. They can also help with headaches, isn't that cool?!

As for probiotics, I am open about my recommendation for Dr. Ohhira's Probiotic because it helps you grow your own intestinal flora, the one you were born with, and plus, it's guaranteed to be alive and fresh. I have recently become a member of their Scientific Advisory board. I've put together a list of popular medications and conditions are among the worst offenders for mugging beneficial bacteria, but bear in mind that if you're taking a drug orally, chances are good it is reducing your garden of healthy bacteria:

Antibiotics
Corticosteroids
Antacids and Acid blockers
Estrogens (birth control and hormone replacement)
Blood pressure pills
Alcohol, even wine

Caffeine-containing drinks
Sugar and refined foods
Having an appendectomy
Celiac, Crohn's and Irritable Bowel Syndrome (IBS)

Pyridoxal 5' Phosphate or P5P

This is an active form of vitamin B6. Not everyone who takes good old B6 can convert it to this biologically active (usable) form of B6. So think of P5P as high-quality B6, a version that works! A deficiency of this B vitamin can make your immune system more likely to attack your thyroid. Also, you need P5P to work with the mineral zinc, which is necessary to make thyroid hormone work. Low levels of this are also associated with premenstrual difficulties, or very bad PMS. A deficiency of P5P in and of itself, can lead to hypothyroidism and more autoimmune thyroid disease. Symptoms of B6 deficiency include depression, irritability and nerve pain. Another possible symptom of B6 deficiency is inflammation of the tongue. You can get inflammation of the tongue with hypothyroidism too, it's almost a hallmark symptom. You can tell if you have this easily, just stick your tongue out. Look in the mirror, does it have mottling on the borders or scalloped edges? This means it is pushing against your teeth because it is bigger than normal. B6 and/or thyroid medication/supplements can help.

Methylcobalamin

This is one of the active forms of vitamin B12. It is not the same as cyanocobalamin, which is an extremely popular, less expensive version of the real deal. Methylcobalamin is what your body utilizes. B12 is a vitamin which has a key role in cell metabolism of your entire body, giving you energy, sharpness in your brain, and healthy nervous system functioning. If you have hypothyroidism, you likely have digestive issues, therefore you could be low in B12.

Some people just cannot recover from thyroid deficiencies even if you give them straight T3 medications. Recent data suggests the reason for this could be B12 deficiency. You see, B12 deficiency goes hand in hand with hypothyroidism. A 2008 study published in *The Journal of the Pakistan Medical Association* evaluated 116 patients suffering from hypothyroidism. The researchers found that almost 40% of hypothyroid patients also suffered with B12 deficiency, that's almost half of you!

Taking B12 with your thyroid hormone replacement medications or supplements should be okay, but you can also ask your health care practitioner.

And having low B12 can affect how much thyroid hormone you make, it's a vicious circle. An animal study that showed B12 deficiency slightly reduces 5' deiodinase activity in the liver, resulting in a significant reduction of T3 (active thyroid hormone) in the tissues. Can we assume the same peripheral reduction in thyroid hormone occurs in humans too? It's not conclusive, but I am betting it does.

One more thing, if you have high homocysteine, a small study found that it could be correlated with hypothyroidism (*Annals of Internal Medicine* 1999). A few months after taking thyroid medication, the patients homocysteine levels came into normal range. So if you think B12 is not important to your thyroid health, please reconsider.

Iodine

Low iodine makes you tired and makes it harder to handle stress. You start to feel fuzzy in the head, get bad PMS and feel slightly depressed. You need iodine to make thyroid hormone, it is part of the backbone of thyroxine (T4). I've discussed this in depth, earlier in this book. Not only is iodine important to making thyroid hormone, it's also needed to protect the reproductive organs, and it may be useful for fibrocystic breast pain. I am somewhat conservative about iodine, I love the trace mineral but only in small, healthy amounts, and only if you are low according to urine tests (skin patch tests aren't reliable).

Remember, in my book, thyroid disease is due to inflammation, not iodine deficiency! If you have poor production of T4, this could be due to iodine deficiency since iodine is needed to make T4.

You can easily become iodine deficient. We are bombarded daily. Halide molecules such as fluorine, chlorine and bromine compete for the same receptor site (the same spot on the cell) as iodine and will win entry into your cell over iodine. Reducing fluorine, chlorine and bromine can help. Read Chapter 8, *Thyroid Thieves Lurking Everywhere.* There are unsuspecting ways we get these thyroid killers into our body:

Taking a shower without a chlorine filter attached
Swimming in a pool or hot tub (chlorine)
Brushing your teeth with fluoride toothpaste
Drinking tap water because it could be
     fluorinated/chlorinated
Breathing in the 'new car' smell, it's off-gassing of bromide
Drinking certain popular power or electrolyte drinks
Cooking with "brominated" vegetable oil
Eating a bagel
Fluoroquinolone antibiotics (Levaquin, Cipro, Avelox)
SSRI antidepressants (Prozac, Paxil, etc)

Zinc

Zinc is critical to activate T4 to T3 in the liver and kidneys. It does that by improving the function of those D (deiodinase) enzymes that activate thyroid hormone. An animal study showed that zinc deficiency strongly reduces activity of this enzyme by up to 67%. If you reduce activity of the enzyme that wakes you up, you are going to feel tired and hypothyroid.

According to a human study, zinc supplementation was able to reestablish normal thyroid function in hypothyroid patients (who were being treated with anticonvulsants like phenytoin or carbamazepine). In another study nine of thirteen participants with low Free T3 (but normal T4) had mild to moderate zinc deficiency. After oral supplementation with zinc sulfate (dosage range was 4-10 mg/kg body weight for 12 months), the levels of serum Free T3 and T3 normalized, rT3 decreased which is a good thing, and TSH normalized. The amount of zinc you have on board influences peripheral metabolism of thyroid hormones and specifically activation of T4 to T3.

Selenium

Selenium helps with thyroid hormone production and usage. More specifically, this antioxidant mineral is essential for the D (deiodinase) enzyme which converts T4 to T3. Deficiency of selenium equates to lower T3 levels. In essence, it means you could be clinically hypothyroid even though circulating levels of T3 and T4 are normal on your lab. Selenium is also needed to balance excess thyroid activity that may be caused by external or internal stressors. Selenium deficiency can also increase hibernation rT3 levels. Selenium protects your thyroid gland from damage from excessive iodine exposure. It's often used in Hashimoto's disease, but it's ideally taken after you have normalized your iodine levels, not before that.

Selenium is truly remarkable when it comes to autoimmune thyroid disease like Hashi's. A clinical trial evaluated patients for 9 months, and concluded that selenium supplementation reduced thyroid peroxidase (TPO) antibody levels in the blood, even in selenium sufficient patients. Remember that TPO antibodies attack your thyroid and cause autoimmune disease (Hashimoto's). Probably 80% of hypothyroid patients have Hashimoto's whether they know it or not.

If you have Hashi's or Graves' I would beg you to get a little selenium approved by your physician (it's sold without prescription but of course I always want you to gain your practitioner's blessings for dietary supplements). Many studies show it can significantly reduce inflammatory cytokines. Remember how I explained to you that inflammation causes your thyroid hormone to become lazy? Selenium helps unlock the door to your cells so your thyroid hormone can get inside the house and turn on the lights and power.

Reducing inflammation is key to preventing more damage to your thyroid tissue and to waking it up. Foods that reduce inflammation (due to being high in selenium are perfect thyroid foods). Selenium works, but how you ask? Scientists suspect this happens (in part), due to the increase in glutathione production. There is also a reduction in toxic free radicals like hydrogen peroxide and lipid hydroperoxides.

Manganese

You need manganese to form the most potent antioxidant you have called "Superoxide Dismutase" and super it is! This enzyme is critical to your mitochondria, which make energy for you, and wake you up. The mitochondria convert glucose into energy by spawning ATP, our energy. Think of ATP as the spark of life generated by these mitochondria. I called them "powerhouses" in my *Diabetes without Drugs* book because they generate power for you. Thyroid hormone doesn't work unless your mitochondria are alive and thriving. As it pertains to thyroid health, this enzyme (which is dependent on manganese) is the primary antioxidant and protector of thyroid hormone in your liver!

Most T4 to T3 conversion occurs in cells from your the liver, so protecting those cells is of utmost importance. As an added benefit, manganese helps people who are "pear-shaped" because it's useful in fat metabolism. It specifically helps reduce fat accumulation in the liver which can cause lipid peroxides! Those compounds tend to put more fat on your hips and thighs.

Controlling the production of fat accumulation in the liver (which is what manganese does) makes it your anti-pear mineral.

Indirectly, it may control sweet cravings. A little manganese is okay like when you see this on the label of your multivitamin or thyroid supplement. It's there for a reason because it works in tandem with other nutrients and minerals to improve brain chemistry. I don't want you to buy a stand alone formula and manganese all by itself, but I suggest lower doses, like when you see it on the label included in a multi-tasking formula. That should be just fine. You can eat some by including salads, green leafy vegetables in your diet, as well as nuts, seeds, molasses, summer squash, strawberries, garlic, hummus, cloves, cinnamon, peppermint and thyme.

Molybdenum

You need molybdenum to convert sulfites in your meals, dried fruit, wine and sulfur-containing foods (like broccoli, garlic, onions) into sulfate. Some people have a genetic mutation or snp (pronounced snip) causing them difficulty in making this conversion. The enzyme that makes this conversion is called "sulfite oxidase." Minimizing sulfur-containing foods will help, and taking very small amounts of molybdenum could too. Another enzyme which helps reduce that 'drunk' feeling in the head is aldehyde oxidase, and it also requires molybdenum.

People with brain fog, or poor concentration may have molybdenum deficiencies. Also, there are other clues such as having asthma, crackly joints, sensitivity to aspirin and salicylates, dislike of sulfur foods, including eggs, arthritis, and emotional problems related to depression (which could be a sign of low dopamine).

Ashwagandha

Known botanically as Withania somnifera, this is an incredible herb. It's intelligent and helps you adapt, that's why it's called an "adaptogen" and it stimulates production of thyroid hormones (T4 and T3) in your body. It also helps nourish your adrenal glands, so if you feel like you can't cope, this is a wonderful botanical to consider. It could help if you feel up or down. Ashwagandha may help reduce swelling (inflammation), regulate blood pressure and improve immunity.

It supports thyroid and adrenal health, so keep this one close to your heart. In fact, I often suggest it as an option for people who can't tolerate the T4 drugs such as Levothyroxine (one brand is Synthroid). You see, ashwagandha has the ability to help hyper and hypo thyroid. It sometimes poses a problem for Hashimoto's patients though. In hypothyroid people, it helps you make more thyroid hormone. It nourishes those poor, tired adrenals that you've burnt out from taking care of a loved one, or from watching *The Tonight Show* instead of sleeping. So ashwagandha (and selenium) are two rock stars when it comes to improving the health of your thyroid gland, and protecting it from DNA damage (which leads to cancer sometimes). Ashwagandha (and selenium) have both been shown to have anti-inflammatory and anti-tu-morigenic effects.

Resveratrol

Well known for its ability to protect the heart, pancreas and brain, resveratrol (Polygonum root) turns on your life-extension gene, called SIRT1 (silent information regulator 1), dubbed the "skinny gene."

I have pages on this antioxidant in my *Diabetes Without Drugs* book because it is so amazing. Some people with Lyme disease use it to control Bartonella organisms. As for thyroid function, resveratrol may help prevent or slow growth of both papillary and follicular thyroid cancer. It causes cancer cells to commit suicide, so there are less of them in your body. Resveratrol enhances iodine utilization, metabolism and thyroid function by affecting SIRT1 gene, and many others. Speaking of cancer, thyroid cancer is on the rise, especially children who have been affected by Fukushima radiation from Japan.

Tyrosine. This is an amino acid (protein building block), which is essential to making thyroid hormone, it combines with iodine to make T4 from your thyroid gland. Tyrosine is vital to making happy brain chemicals and neurotransmitters such as L-dopa, dopamine, epinephrine and norepinephrine. So critical is tyrosine that without it, you will become moody, tired and hypothyroid. Apart from its critical role in people who have hypothyroidism, tyrosine can be important to those with depression, Parkinson's disease, addiction and alcohol withdrawal support. A cool tidbit about tyrosine is that it's converted into melanin by your skin cells, and melanin helps you tan, plus, it helps protect you from harmful UV (ultraviolet) light.

Lots of healthcare practitioners suggest high doses of tyrosine, such as 500 mg two or three times daily, but I do not agree. While it's a great precursor to thyroid hormone, I think a little does the body just fine. Remember, thyroid disease is (in my book) a disease of inflammatory chemicals running amok, and also adequate thyroid hormone that can no longer get inside your cells. I'm more interested in making your thyroid hormone work for you (get it inside your cells, and if you recall my original analogy, I want to get it inside your house to turn the light and power on), than I am pumping you full of more thyroid hormone that is essentially useless because you can't use it. So "yes" to tyrosine, but not big doses or it can stimulate you too much, inducing high blood pressure, headaches, sleep disturbances, insomnia and cardiac palpitations. High doses of tyrosine (like 500mg and above per day) should not be taken with thyroid medications, as far as I'm concerned; lower doses however, are usually okay but always ask your practitioner what is right for you. I can't possibly know how you'll personally react to any supplement I educate you on.

Mullein. This herb is known botanically as "Verbascum thapsus" and has strong medicinal benefits and antibiotic actions against tuberculosis, leprosy and many other pathogens. It is a strong anti-infectious herb which is a big deal to me because we are all toting bugs around in our body, it's a question of when they become opportunistic. Mullein grows like a weed in open pastures where I live in Colorado and if you've ever gone on a hike, I know you've seen one of the varieties with yellow flowers. One plant can generate 100,000 seeds in a year that are capable of surviving for 100 years! This resilient plant has activity against some of the world's worst pathogens. Furthermore, mullein possesses strong anti-inflammatory, anti-tumor, antifungal, antibacterial and anti-viral actions. Herbalists and holistic practitioners use it sometimes as an expectorant because it reduces congestion in the lungs. It has analgesic properties from its healing polysaccharides and flavonoids which reduce inflammatory cytokines (by blocking NF-kB, a pathway in your body that churns pain-causing compounds). Because of its ability to reduce superoxide free radicals, it could reduce glandular inflammation associated with Graves' disease or Hashimoto's. This herb can be purchased all by itself as a stand alone, and it's also in ThyroScript, a formula I custom made. I want you to discuss taking all supplements with your doctor, even if they are naturally amazing.

Part VI
Getting Thyroid Healthy

Chapter 20

Foods That Heal Your Thyroid

What you eat can affect your thyroid gland in a critical way. This chapter will highlight some nutrients and foods that support thyroid hormone production and activation. This may be all you need to do to lose a little weight and feel more energetic. If it's not, you can always ask your doctor about taking supplements and/or medications. First up is iodine, because that's what your thyroid gland needs to make thyroxine (T4).

Iodine. Iodine is a trace element and one that your thyroid must have to create the hormone in the first place. Deficiency of iodine used to be rare in the United States, but a recent figure from the *Centers for Disease Control* (CDC) reveals Americans are becoming increasingly iodine deficient. I don't think we should be supplementing with huge doses indefinitely but I also think that many experts are iodine-phobic. Many people are deficient in iodine because they take SSRI antidepressants for a long time, or they drink tap water. It's easy to become deficient. Getting iodine from foods is pretty easy, and when you can't, you can also supplement. There is much more on iodine in Chapter 20, *Foods That Heal Your Thyroid*. Iodine deficiency is one leading cause of hypothyroidism worldwide and it is a risk factor for thyroid cancer. Low iodine can cause a goiter. Be careful though, there is an article I read recently that suggests an "overdiagnosis" of thyroid cancer when you get imaging done on your neck for goiters. It may or may not be cancer, I'm just saying to get a second opinion if you're given this diagnosis after a neck imaging study. Many experts think that eating "iodized" table salt provides enough iodine. I'm not one of those experts that feels this way. With the exception of iodine, common white table salt is stripped of every single mineral you need to make, absorb and utilize thyroid hormone. Besides that, it's subjected to bleach to give it a white appearance. This leaves a backbone structure of salt called "sodium chloride" which is a chemical in my book, it is not 'food' for your thyroid gland. Think of it that way every time you see a salt shaker at a restaurant because in the final analysis, it's still "sodium chloride," a nutritionally naked salt.

Will Table Salt Give Me Enough Iodine?

Both sea salt and table salt have a backbone of "sodium chloride" which the body requires. Healthy sea salts are never adulterated like regular table salt, so they retain healthy minerals like copper, iodine, potassium, magnesium, chromium, zinc, iron and others. Table salt is so refined that I consider it a food additive because certain brands look virtually like the same industrial chemical used to de-ice highways. No kidding. Sea salt, on the other hand, is not synthesized in a lab. It is essentially water from a sea (or river) that gets evaporated and purified. You can buy these at health food stores, Whole Foods or online. You want your salt to have some color to it. Sea salt is still refined to some extent you know, so I'm asking you to get salt with color.

1. Himalayan salt. When it's mined properly from pristine salt veins in the Himalayan Mountains in Pakistan, it contains the widest variety of minerals, over 83 kinds of minerals. Good Himalayan salt will look slightly pink because it contains a lot of iron. About 1 gram of Himalayan salt has 500 mcg iodine.

2. Celtic sea salt or French Grey Sea Salt. This salt does not have quite as many different minerals in it as the Himalayan sort, however, it has the highest content (gram for gram) of minerals.

3. "Real" salt, by Redmond. I think that is extremely pure and it contains 60 trace minerals. The company gives my fans a 20% discount if you use coupon code "suzycohen" at their site, realsalt.com

It's impossible to get nutritious minerals from typical white table salt and yet people debate this with me pointing out that their salt is healthy because it has been "iodized." Yeah, so what? Someone decided to put iodine back in after stripping it naked in the first place? This is your idea of healthy? You are more likely to be able to lick your elbow than to get thyroid-loving nutrients from white table salt!

Iodine is very good for you, but the amount of table salt you'd have to ingest in order to get healthy amounts of iodine would probably be the end of you! I'm just saying to stop rationalizing the use of table salt, because it provides iodine. I'm also saying that you can't lick your elbow!

Foods Rich in Iodine

Sea vegetables are the richest source, like sea weed. Health-food stores carry a variety of seaweed, in dried or powdered form, such as kelp, dulse flakes (which taste very salty), and kombu. Kelp is one of the world's richest sources of iodine. Dried seaweed makes a nice snack or you can add it or the powdered variation to soups, salads and beans. Salmon skin hand roll anyone? I love those, that is one quick way to crank up your iodine levels because of the seafood and the seaweed wrapped up into one edible package, lip-smacking if you dunk it in spicy mayo!

+ You can make a kelp shaker (similar to a salt shaker); learn how to do that in the spirulina section coming up next.

+ Hawaiian spirulina is an excellent source of iodine. You
  can buy the powder form of spirulina, and put it in a salt
  shaker. It tastes very sulfur-ish (that is the healing
  quality though, the stronger the flavor, the more potent
  your supplement is, meaning good quality). Some
  people crave the flavor, but if it's too sulfur-like for you,
  mix a small amount of spirulina in a shaker with garlic
  powder, onion powder, salt or any spice blend you use
  frequently. You are making your own shaker that way.
  You can combine it into any seasoning that you love, so
  with every shake, you get a small amount of spirulina in
  your food.

  Spirulina is a very rich source of iodine. The brand I
  have at home is Hawaiian Spirulina by Nutrex Hawaii.
  As a side benefit, spirulina is known to chelate heavy
  metals and provide a vegetarian source of protein, B
  vitamins and minerals which you need for total body
  health. They give my fans 25% off with the coupon code
  "suzy" if you buy at their site nutrex-hawaii.com.
+ Seafood such as herring, salmon, sardines and cod. Get
  wild caught seafood. I happen to love herring, but some
  people don't like the strong flavor. Salmon is a milder
  choice, and it's excellent because it also contains small
  amounts of natural astaxanthin. And then there's cod.
  Cod flavor is low-fat, mild and moist making it
  everyone's favorite. One 3 to 4 ounce serving contains
  approximately 100 mcg iodine.
+ Potato with the peel. Bake it! Make sure it's grown
  organically; a medium potato has about 60 mcg iodine.
+ Cow's milk products like yogurt or milk (if you are not
  allergic, and only buy grass-fed organic milk). I'm not a
  fan of dairy but I know some of you drink and eat it all
  the time. It's good to know that one cup of yogurt has
  about 90 mcg iodine.

+ Turkey breast provides about 30 to 40 mcg of iodine.
+ Cranberries. About a half cup contains 400 mcg of iodine. If you're buying juice, it is going to be quite tart. Be careful and read labels to ensure you are consuming a 'clean' brand free of refined sugar, high fructose corn syrup or artificial sweeteners. It may be better to buy the plain version and sweeten it a little at home with a natural sweetener such as honey, unrefined turbinado sugar, coconut sugar or stevia.

The right amount of iodine can breathe life into you, but excess may cause hyperthyroidism! Iodine supplements are available, and sometimes I recommend those for people who can't consume enough naturally. Use dietary supplements only under a doctor's supervision. Iodine alone does not optimize your thyroid production, you probably need selenium so that's up next.

Foods Rich in Selenium

Selenium is one lovely mineral. It has antioxidant powers. It utilizes nutrients to form thyroid hormone, and optimizes your detoxification pathways. This lowers the chance of poisonous waste building up in the thyroid.

Selenium is so critical to your thyroid health that deficiencies of it put you at risk for thyroid cancer! Boosting intake of selenium foods is good for both hypo and hyperthyroidism. It helps both conditions because selenium reduces inflammation. Selenium is also essential for converting inactive T4 into active T3.

Plant foods have selenium, but the soil in many regions of this country is selenium deficient, which means the crops that grow on it are also deficient. The true selenium leader is the Brazil nut and I recommend you eat those every day, but only 4 nuts, or less. Just one Brazil nut provides up to 100 mcg, nearly twice the daily adult RDA of 55 mcg! Choose your nuts wisely because (depending on where you get them), you could have moldy Brazil nuts. The aspergillus on the nuts may cause you to react, especially if you are very sensitive. Here are selenium-rich foods:

+ Seafood
+ Meats (chicken, lamb, turkey, free range game, etc)
+ Mushrooms such as crimini or shitake
+ Asparagus- okay if it's cooked, broiled or seared.
+ Eggs
+ Spinach
+ Nuts
+ Clams- about 410 mcg in a 1 cup serving!
+ Canned or fresh oysters have about 100 mcg in a serving
+ Raw octopus (is anyone but a whale eating this?!) about 100 mcg per 3 oz serving

Foods Rich in Tyrosine

Tyrosine, an amino acid that helps hormone-producing organs, is also essential for healthy thyroid production; remember both T4 and T3 hormones are tyrosine-based. An added bonus of tyrosine: it is a precursor to the "feel-good" neurotransmitter dopamine. If you are tyrosine deficient that means you are suffering a double-whammy, low thyroid hormone and low dopamine. This can lead to dozens of symptoms including depression and anhedonia.

Depression feels different if you're low in serotonin, versus dopamine. This is very general, but if your depression is low serotonin, you crave sweets, carbs, dairy, bananas, you feel hollow inside and you have insomnia.

With low dopamine depression, you crave chocolate, coffee, there's no pleasure or passion, "I just don't care" feeling. It bugs me that physicians presume it's low serotonin and prescribe SSRI antidepressants which increase serotonin. Such drugs include sertraline (Zoloft), fluoxetine (Prozac) and others, but I'm saying these drugs don't help you if your depression is related to low dopamine. This is often the case! You can measure urine levels of dopamine's metabolite called "homovanillate" (some labs call it HVA) to get a better indication of dopamine status; you can also gauge your personal attitude and degree of apathy. And remember, if you are tyrosine deficient, you're not only low in dopamine (depression), you can be hypothyroid too causing dozens of other symptoms. Tyrosine is the backbone of thyroid hormone, as well as dopamine. Tyrosine deficiency can happen easily if you eat the standard American diet (SAD diet) filled with junk food and fast food. It'll definitely make you sad by depleting your iodine and tyrosine over time.

It's important to have plenty of foods with tyrosine in your diet and you can get it from eating protein of all sorts, game meats, poultry, fish, steak, and eggs. Some excellent vegan sources include avocados, banana's and pumpkin seeds. Here are some other rich food sources of tyrosine that can wake up your thyroid:

+ Duck
+ Fava Beans
+ Eggs, specifically the egg white
+ Hawaiian spirulina
+ Kidney beans
+ Mustard greens, spinach and other greens
+ Seafood (orange roughy, tilapia, salmon, haddock, crustaceans, etc)
+ Seaweed like wakame
+ Sesame seeds

Foods Rich in Zinc

Zinc is a trace mineral that functions in 300 metabolic processes in the body. Not surprisingly it's imperative for healthy thyroid function. It's needed to help activate your energy-producing T3. Also, your hypothalamus needs zinc to send it's own signals. Zinc plays a role in blood clotting, reproductive health, prostate health, your senses of hearing, smell and vision. You need zinc to heal your skin so people with poor wound healing need to think about zinc replenishment. Oftentimes, people with zinc deficiency have hair loss, or hair thinning, poor hearing, reduced sense of smell, low appetite, symptoms of hypothyroidism, prostate enlargement, fertility problems and/or white spots on the fingernails. Read Chapter 23, *Solutions for Thyroid Symptoms*, for solutions to some of these problems.

A 2007 study published in the *Annals of Nutrition and Metabolism* found that young women could boost conversion of T3 (from T4) by taking about 26 mg zinc gluconate supplements for several months. Many studies confirm zinc's importance to your metabolism. Careful though, supplementing can backfire sometimes, like if you take too much. For example, zinc supplementation can reduce iron in the body, and then your "ferritin" will become reduced. Ferritin is a stored form of iron that is measurable with a blood test. Low ferritin means you are very tired, pale and short of breath and that's the tip of the iceberg. I had low ferritin for years, but now it is normal and I feel the difference in energy and endurance.

High amounts of zinc can cause a copper deficiency, which in turn can lead to a wide variety of health problems including excessive T4 in the bloodstream. This triggers a thyroid 'situation' where your thyroid has to work harder, and you may feel clinically hypothyroid. Now you see why I'm all about food! Eating foods rich in zinc is my preference rather than taking supplements which can backfire. It's hard to eat too much zinc. You should only take supplements if you need them, and you are supervised by a knowledgable practitioner.

Vegetarians often have more serious zinc deficiencies than others, and require higher supplement doses than protein lovers. Eating a diet that includes lean red meats can help increase the levels of zinc. However, in many well-developed countries where health conscious individuals shun red meats, zinc deficiency is common. There are hundreds of drug muggers of zinc, among the most common are estrogen containing medications, corticosteroids, certain cholesterol binding drugs, antacids and acid blockers. A complete list of drugs that zap zinc from your body (and compromise thyroid function) is found in my *Drug Muggers* book.

People with gastrointestinal diseases are also more susceptible to zinc deficiency, and therefore thyroid dysfunction. You may benefit from a little bit of zinc if you:

+ Have conditions that affect your brain (epilepsy, schizophrenia, obsessive compulsive)
+ Have an eating disorder (anorexia or bulimia)
+ If you drink alcohol or coffee
+ If you fail to ovulate properly, or don't get a regular period
+ If you have sickle cell anemia, Celiac disease or Irritable Bowel Syndrome
+ If you have kidney disease
+ If you have diabetes

Alcoholics have a real hard time keeping zinc on board. They are about 50% more likely to have a zinc deficiency due to their reduced ability to absorb nutrients; plus, they have increased urination which causes them to eliminate zinc faster. Here are some foods that are rich in zinc:

+ Oysters have a lot of zinc, it's incredible, about 60 to 120 mg natural zinc per 3 ounce serving, so this is your richest source. It's okay to cook/steam them.
+ Cereals are great sources of zinc, but I do not recommend you eat popular supermarket cereals, they almost always contain gluten and grains which can increase autoimmune types of thyroid disease. I will elaborate on this more very soon.
+ Miso soup, just make sure it does not have MSG and too much sodium.

✦ Spices such as freeze-dried parsley and chives; both of these contain about 6 mg of zinc per tablespoon. If you sprinkle it into your soup at the end of cooking, you'll have a tasty addition of flavor to go with the zinc.

✦ Pumpkin seeds are fabulous, even raw and you can roast them with a little garlic, salt and grape seed oil. Craveable!

✦ Dried Shitake mushrooms have many other medicinal benefits. You can 'wet' them by soaking in pure water, or adding to soup. About 8 mg zinc for a handful.

✦ Sesame butter or Tahini- About 10mg per serving.

✦ Watermelon seed kernels- Say what? Yes, it's true. You can buy dried "watermelon seed kernels" and you can gnash on them like you would pumpkin seeds, you can also grind a few into your smoothie. There's about 5 mg in half a cup. Seafood- all kinds of seafood, including crustaceans like lobster, shrimp, etc.

✦ Sunflower seeds or sunflower butter is an excellent way to get zinc! Eat the seeds, or spread the sunflower butter on celery or apples... or put some butter in your smoothie.

✦ Nuts, especially Brazil nuts, pine nuts, pecans, almonds and walnuts. Make sure you buy organic, pesticides attack your thyroid gland. You may want to peel the skin on the almonds (to do that soak them in water for 4 hours, then squeeze them out of their skin).

Coconut Oil

Long viewed as a "bad" fat, coconut oil has recovered its reputation as fat that is healthy and good for you. Coconut oil is often called thyroid-friendly for those with hypothyroidism and the low metabolism that it causes. The reason is that this oil is made up primarily of medium-chain fatty acids, as opposed to the long-chain fatty acids of most oils. Medium-chain fatty acids increase metabolism because they are small enough to directly enter the cell's mitochondria, where cells convert the fatty acids into energy.

Vegetable oils that contain anything "brominated" on the label can harm the thyroid gland by displacing iodine and reducing your ability to make thyroid hormone. So coconut oil is a great substitute, and it has a high smoke point unlike olive oil. You can cook with coconut oil, put it in smoothies, or even swallow a tablespoon of it plain. Coconut oil on your skin can be divine, many people with hypothyroid suffer with dry skin, a hallmark sign of sluggish thyroid. One of the active ingredients in coconut oil is monolaurin, which helps reduce inflammation while also revving up thyroid hormone production. I like coconut "butter" too, it's fabulous to put in smoothies, and sometimes I've been known to spoon it on a cracker.

Vitamin A

You need vitamin A to make your thyroid work well. Eat sweet potatoes, butternut squash and cantaloupes. Zinc works in tandem with vitamin A, and both support thyroid health and vision.

Chapter 21

Foods That Can Keep You "Thyroid Sick"

Let's talk about foods and beverages that could possibly harm you. You will likely be surprised to learn that for those of you with hypothyroidism, one category of bad-for-you foods are super-healthy for most people. I'm referring to cruciferous vegetables (also called brassica), which includes nutritional power-houses as broccoli, mustard greens and cauliflower.

Cruciferous vegetables are okay in moderation and I still recommend you eat them. But if you eat a lot, such as more than 5 servings per week, it may become a problem because they are considered goitrogens, which means they interfere with the uptake of iodine by your thyroid gland. A reduced supply of iodine, as we have seen, suppresses production of thyroid hormone. Goitrogens also can cause an enlargement of the thyroid, called a goiter by reducing iodine. Goitrogen foods includ broccoli, Brussels sprouts, cabbage, cauliflower, kale, kohlrabi, rutabaga, and turnips. If you eat a truckload, over time these foods can cause a goiter, or enlargement of the thyroid gland. There's controversy about cooking these foods, and if that inactivates goitrogenic compounds, personally I think cooked goitrogens are fine, in moderation.

Soy

Soy is a legume. There is much controversy surrounding it. If you ask me, I would say avoid it. I'm aware of the controversy, we have many health experts touting it as a cure-all for many conditions, most notably, menopause. And then other experts, like my friend Dr. Joseph Mercola (*Mercola.com*) pointing out the health concerns, and the genetically modified problems that most soy has. I personally think soy-based foods, especially in excess can be harmful to the thyroid because they are strong goitrogens and it's true, soy is often genetically modified or GMO. That's not to say that once a year I don't eat edamame beans with a little salt on them, but hey that's really rare. I know people who live on soy diets and they don't look well, or feel well. Soy foods are often heavily processed (think soy milk), and so I feel they are best avoided or kept to a minimum. Soy-based meals like turkey made of soy, or soy cheese are what I affectionately call "fake plastic food." For me, and I know this is a touchy subject, but I just don't like "cheese" that has 20 ingredients, or "turkey" that has like 40 ingredients. This is not healthy in my opinion, you're better off taking the dairy hit and eating real cheese, and likewise, eating turkey, it's just one ingredient, turkey!

Gluten

Celiac is the autoimmune condition where your body reacts to certain proteins like those in gluten (wheat). The most shocking thing is that only 50% of people tested for Celiac disease ever come up positive, the rest of you that actually have this auto-immune disease will be told you're fine. The reason is because for decades, standard blood tests only checked for "alpha" gliadin, but that is just one sub-unit of the entire gluten protein. What if you are not allergic to alpha, but you are severely allergic to the omega, gamma, or glutenin portion of the molecule?

You will be told that it's safe to continue eating wheat (gluten) and this will continue to damage your thyroid gland. You may stay locked in sickness, because doctors testing for gluten sensitivity, or for that matter all food sensitivities are almost always using standard labs instead of specialized ones that use state-of-the-art equipment to find sensitivities to all portions of the gluten molecule. The big shocker here is that people who are allergic to gluten, are almost always also allergic to other grains as well as dairy. I hear you already, what's left to eat! Plenty, I assure you. The lab I recommend for food sensitivity testing is Cyrex Labs.

Studies have shown that gluten foods (wheat, rye, barley) have a strong connection to both Hashimoto's disease and Graves' disease. The explanation is a curious scenario. The molecular structure of the protein in gluten closely resembles that of the thyroid gland. Sometimes gluten molecules slip past the gut barrier, making their way into the blood stream, and this is where it gets really interesting. The gliadin proteins (these are the smaller parts of gluten) love your thyroid gland, so they go and hang out over there, in your thyroid tissue. Bad news! The body's immune system sees these gliadin (and other gluten-related proteins) as invaders and goes after them. Well, why not? That's its job, to go after foreign looking antigens, in this case gliadin, glutenin and other gluten-related proteins. Your immune system attacks the thyroid tissue.

The point is, because of the similarity in structure, the thyroid gland become collateral damage by your own immune system because that is where the gluten goes!

If you have Hashi's I urge you to go grain free, or at the very least, gluten free. That is definitely my preference, grain free! But even if you try eating meals free of gluten I'd be happy. Researchers have shown the connection repeatedly. By connection, I mean auto-immune thyroid disease connected to anti-gliadin antibodies (gluten sensitivity). Read more about Hashimoto's in Chapter 17.

People with thyroid illness commonly have migraines. Gluten is what I call a migrenade™ in my "Headache Free" book because when you eat it, it seems to spark a headache or migraine in susceptible individuals. Eating gluten free could speed healing for thyroid illness and migraines all in one fell swoop. Trust me when I tell you, your thyroid gland and your brain responds happily for you if you cut out gluten. Celiac often goes hand in hand with thyroid disease. I've seen the diet reduce TPO antibodies in my friend by 75% in just 2 months of a strict gluten free diet. To that end, a study published in the *Journal of Clinical Endocrinology and Metabolism*, states, "Malabsorption of T4 may provide the opportunity to detect Celiac Disease that was overlooked until the patients were put under T4 therapy."

You can do a saliva test and find out if you have the Celiac gene. I tested myself using 23andMe.com and found out I have this gene, however, I do not have Celiac, nor any backlash from eating gluten. It's because I rarely get into gluten, maybe occasionally when traveling. My diet goes to pot when I travel honestly. Nevertheless, I choose to remain gluten free for general health purposes. Try it for 60 to 90 days, and then evaluate your symptoms and your response to thyroid medication. Maybe you'll be able to reduce medication dosage if you're strict about your new meal plan.

Complete avoidance of grains is known to reduce antibodies in your body, especially those directed at your thyroid gland. Does your body digest gluten on its own? Yes, it does to some extent, but gluten is a food additive, it's not really natural like you think it is. Think of it in the same way you do MSG or artificial colors, it's an additive like that. It's not necessary, not even for taste. It's there to hold stuff together, like glue. Maybe they should have spelled it "glue-ten" instead of "gluten."

This is pretty cool: Your body has its own digestive enzyme for gluten called "dipeptidyl peptidase-IV" or DPPIV. You make that.

Some people have a deficiency in this enzyme, therefore you have trouble breaking down the protein. Partial digestion of the gluten protein can exasperate your gastrointestinal tract, inflame the small intestine, and thus launch an immune response which attacks your thyroid gland. Remember what I told you about inflammation? It's bad for your thyroid gland. Gluten causes the release of inflammatory cytokines. There's good news.

You can take supplements that contain "DPPIV" and this gives you an edge in digesting the gluten. The enzyme DPPIV stands for "dipeptidyl peptidase four" and it may offer some protection to your thyroid gland if you do happen to eat gluten. DPPIV (pronounced DPP four) blocks gluten absorption to some degree, but it doesn't block it all. One such supplement is Gluten-Ease™ by Enzymedica. The dietary supplement I formulated called Thyro-Script contains this enzyme, plus nutrients that support thyroid health and healthy metabolism. I don't let others sell it, so it's only available at my site *www.ScriptEssentials.com*. By the way, I have another site where you can read articles about other health topics, *www.SuzyCohen.com*.

DPPIV is intended to protect your body from gluten, but it can't neutralize 100% of the gluten you eat. Some of the gluten you consume is still going to get absorbed, the enzyme just assists you. I recommend that you eat gluten free, and preferably grain free while taking ThyroScript however this diet is not absolutely necessary for my supplement to help you.

If you have either type of autoimmune thyroid illness (Hashi's or Graves') then please avoid gluten completely. Like I said, people find the most effective results when eating a completely grain free diet. This is called a Paleo diet, or Phase One diet, or sometimes "Hunter Gatherer" diet. There are many websites, books and recipe books devoted to this now. When I was eating a strict Paleo diet (not due to hypothyroidism, but just because of the health benefits), I found that cooking with almond flour was delicious, it's grain free, and it has a nice texture. I buy mine online, however, there are some brands sold at grocery stores.

The important part here, is that gluten has a particularly strong affinity for thyroid tissue and has been shown repeatedly in studies to increase antibodies to thyroid, and to bind to both benign and malignant thyroid nodules. Guess what might cause a thyroid nodule? You'll never guess, it's an artificial sweetener called ACE-K or "acesulfame." It's structurally related to a growth hormone, and may cause benign nodules. Now, back to this thyroid nodule problem.

By no means am I advocating you get a thyroid biopsy, you can if you want, but I want you to hear about this Lancet study. Researchers took tired patients and did biopsies on their thyroid. Not even half of them showed inflammation (as in lymphocytic thyroiditis). But they were all treated with thyroid hormone, specifically T3. They all responded, it didn't matter what their TSH was. Remember, TSH is a brain hormone and can be normal even when you're dead tired. So basically, only 40% of those with inflammation, had an abnormal TSH, but they all got better with thyroid hormone replacement. When I'm speaking to doctors or pharmacist peers, I tell them, "You can't go biopsying everyones thyroid! But you can give your patients a thyroid replacement medication and see how they respond." The authors of the Lancet study also say the same thing in their own words, "After treatment with thyroxine, clinical response was favorable, irrespective of baseline TSH concentration."

Thyroid Healthy Tip

Have you been told you have a thyroid nodule? This is a small growth on your thyroid. If your doctor tells you the nodule is "hot" this means it's producing hormones, often in excess. If your nodule is "cold" it means that your low in thyroid hormone, likely from low iodine. Cold nodules are often relieved by administering iodine. Ask your doctor to do an iodine test to assess your levels, the best way to do this is with an overnight (24 hour) urine catch. Many labs can do this including Quest.

Chapter 22

How to Construct a Healthy Kitchen

I'm about to blow the lid off the conventional food pyramid which makes many people sicker. I won't bore you with food cultivation and production techniques, although you should know that our soils are depleted, and supermarkets are filled will plastic fake pharma-foods.

Here's secret #1: Soy can make you sleepy. It attacks the thyroid gland and is a known goitrogen, suppressing thyroid activity. Mothers are feeding their babies soy-based formulas, it's like giving their child the estrogenic equivalent of some birth control pills every morning! Not only does this practice raise estrogen in the human body, it suppresses thyroid hormone production. Yet, there is a big commercial soy push and a myriad of soy formulas offered to young mothers looking for alternatives to breast milk.

Other foods that you consume can also crash your thyroid hormone, take a look:

+ Cabbage
+ Brussels sprouts
+ Cauliflower
+ Broocoli
+ Lima beans

Secret #2: Do you eat the standard American diet? We live in a McThyroid Generation!

Secret #3: Do you drink alcohol or coffee?

Alcohol, food additives, dyes and other chemicals in your meals damage your intestinal lining therefore, they are also gut grenades. A damaged lining allows undigested food particles to leak out, some of which have a protein sequence similar to thyroid tissue, so your thyroid gland accepts these food particles and then your immune system follows suit with an attack. It's only doing what it knows to do, it doesn't realize there is delicate, life-sustaining thyroid tissue there, it's just trying to get rid of those foreign food proteins. Too bad your thyroid can't defend itself.

Secret #4: Gut grenades: Gluten is a major factor, and contributes to chronic inflammation, it's a protein found in wheat, barley, rye and it's a huge offender for thyroid function. Between the genetically-modified foods and proteins, the body says "What's this?" It causes a chronic inflammatory condition in the body, and contributes to the epidemic of thyroid disease.

Other 'Gut Grenades' that lead to Immune Dysregulation:

+ Pollen
+ Plastic
+ Heavy metals (like mercury)
+ Pesticide exposure
+ Medications

It's not what you add, it's what you should eliminate!

+ Plastic tupperware—BPA kills the thyroid gland
+ Cosmetics containing parabens
+ Tuna—the mercury harms thyroid tissue
+ Plastic water bottles
+ White table salt

Only eat pure unrefined salt. You don't want table salt, it is nutritionally naked, and lacks dozens of thyroid-loving minerals. From now on, it's only Himalayan (pink) salt, Celtic Salt or REAL salt.

When I Say Elimination, I Mean Eliminate!

Do you know what happens in your home if you don't take out the trash every day? Same thing with you. In the next section I'll teach you how to effectively clear your bowels gently, and promote optimal intestinal healthy. About 20 percent of thyroid hormone is activated in the gut, and it only requires one thing, probiotic supplements. This rarely discussed fact is common knowledge in my world. The lack of probiotics will tremendously impact your health, from head to toe. Sometimes it's all you need to get well. Did you know an aspirin a day will destroy your probiotic flora? So will 1 cup of coffee, or a glass of wine per day.

Most people with thyroid disorders are overweight. They go on a diet to lose stubborn weight, but if you scramble the word "diet" you get "edit" and that is what I would teach people to do in this chapter. Teaching them to "Edit" what they eat, rather than "Diet" and this could be a life saver for them. In the case of soda pop, which many Americans are addicted to, a simple edit would include my own recipe, which is half a cup of carbonated seltzer water with half a cup of pomegranate or grape juice (or even root-beer flavored stevia drops). It works like a charm, it's all natural, and helps break even years of addictions to soda.

A thyroid-friendly kitchen is critical to healing, and my information will be highly practical and easy to implement. My diet plan, "Foods to Fuel You" will include dishes that are based on the "hunter-gatherer" diet, also termed the Paleo Diet which suggests eliminating all refined foods, sugar, starches, grains and legumes among other things. According to the Paleo way of eating, and I'm really simplifying things here, it is the avoidance of grains that will help normalize thyroid function, as well as blood sugar, appetite, cravings, weight loss and production of energy. There does come a time when one can integrate a few grains in the diet, but not in the beginning.

Marry Me Banana Bread

(My husband jokes with me and says he married me for this bread, I've adapted it because at the time we were both consuming dairy)

2½ cups almond flour
½ cup chopped walnuts
1 tea baking soda
⅛ teaspoon REAL salt
1/2 cup grape seed oil
2 large ripe bananas
1 tablespoon flax seed (ground)
1/2 cup Blue Raw Agave syrup (or organic maple syrup)
1 tea vanilla extract (or banana extract)
2 eggs
Cinnamon
Optional: ¼ cup semi-sweet chocolate chips

Mix together, bake 350 degrees, in a greased 6 x 9 baking dish.

Coconut Oil and Coconut Butter- Eat it every single day. It's a powerful anti-fungal, it can provide the body with medium chain triglycerides (good ones) and it can help energize you. Great for dryness associated with thyroid conditions, you can slather the oil on dry cracked heels, eczema rashes and elbows. Hey, for that matter, condition your hair with a little bit.

The way you cook, and the ingredients you use in your meals hold the key to getting you thyroid healthy. Every meal is an opportunity for success. Food choices become especially important if you have an autoimmune thyroid illness. Pasta becomes an enemy as does anything with pesticides or artificial sweeteners. The pans you use to cook with are important too. And guess what else, that little salt shaker with "table salt" is a problem, it should contain real salt, the kind with a little color. I mean Real™ Salt by Redmond, or an equivalent that has color.

Your dream is to get thin and feel healthy and energetic. Your wish is my command, that's why I've written this next section. It won't be easy to adapt to some of these changes and I understand that. I have confidence in you though, and I believe in time, you'll be able to make some of the changes outlined in this chapter. Every little thing you do will give you some benefit, and after you see some changes, maybe your hair grows faster, or your nails don't break as much, perhaps some weight comes off, or you sleep a little better, maybe energy goes up a little ... at some point you'll trust me and you'll know I've got your back! Then you'll want to do even more and you'll stop thinking this lady is crazy. How do I know that? Because I've written 6 other books on various topics and I get hundreds of 5 star reviews on Amazon and 'love' notes and praise to my email every single day! In the coming pages you'll learn how to help restock your kitchen better and choose wisely while eating out so that you can eat foods that heal your thyroid, rather than harm it. You only have one precious thyroid gland, and it's delicate. Remember, it's a butterfly shaped gland so you can easily think about it like a butterfly. They're wings are thin, and very delicate. Allow me to ask you a few personal questions. It will help you identify the problem areas of your kitchen and cabinets. My goal is to help you clean it out now, so you can restock it with safer, healthier choices.

Question 1: What Oils Do You Use?

Commercial hormone-laden heavily refined cheese, butter and oils may increase thyroid cancer risk! I know you are hearing how lately these things are good for you but I'm not a fan of them, unless they are from grass-fed animals raised without antibiotics or hormones. You have to understand that the fat tissues of an animal collect all the garbage and poisons that animal eats or gets exposed to. These toxins hide in the fat, so if you're eating concentrated fatty oils from these animals they better be from clean animals not commercial ones. I mention the virtues of coconut oil as frequently as possible. I also highly recommend olive oil, tea seed and grape seed oil, as alternatives to butter. Ghee is fine if it's the absolute highest quality clean ghee. I think cheese is best avoided or at least minimized. I know you want to live a little so please enjoy it, but as infrequently as possible. My conversation is aimed at people who have cheese and butter with bread, literally for breakfast lunch and dinner, every day. I'm not worried if you indulge once or twice a week for example. Goat cheese is fine once in a while, but not the kind that is cow-derived as in "feta" I'm okay with pure goat cheese at times, in moderation.

My comments are based on pooled clinical data completed in Europe that found consumption of cheese, butter and certain oils correlated to thyroid disease and cancer. The scientists looked at 385 histologically confirmed (real, authentic) cases of thyroid cancer and compared them to almost 800 controls (people without thyroid cancer). There was a direct and significant association between thyroid cancer patients consuming more starchy foods (ie bread, pastries ... hmm, could it have been gluten? I suspect), potatoes, cheese and butter. There was an inverse correlation (that's good in this case) with participants who ate carrots, green salads and citrus fruits. You think that was a fluke? No it was not, the scientists even concluded, "These results were consistent and reproducible across various study centers." So the oils you choose to put in your salad, and cook with have an impact on your thyroid gland. Get the harmful ones out of your kitchen.

Question #2: Do You Eat Whole Grains?

You shouldn't. Italian researchers who examined data over 13 years, concluded in 1998 that a diet rich in whole grain foods was harmful to your thyroid. High intake of whole grain foods consistently reduced the risk of tumors everywhere in the body except the thyroid. The take-home point is that whole grains hurt the thyroid. Current research suggests whole grains aggravate thyroid conditions, especially Graves' and Hashimoto's. Experts today frequently recommend a grain-free (Paleo) diet. When baking, substitute all-purpose (wheat flour) for almond, coconut, hemp or chickpea. Most of you will do fine with rice flour, despite it being a grain.

Question #3: What Are You Cooking In?

Chances are good that you have non-stick pans in your kitchen. I know I do, but I use it no more than twice a year, at very low temperatures. After reading the following you may want to buy new pots and pans. Here's why: a large study investigated a link between thyroid disease and exposure to PFOA (perfluorooctanoic acid), an organic chemical used in many products. The study found that people with the highest PFOA concentration in their blood were twice as likely to have thyroid disease as those with the lowest levels. No one knows exactly why, but experts surmise that the PFOA may disrupt binding of thyroid hormones, or it might interfere with metabolism or activation of the hormones in the liver. Some better choices would be stainless steel or cast iron.

Question #4: Do You Choose Organic Foods Whenever Possible?

You are going to have to fight for your thyroid health. We live in a world where hundreds of thousands of chemicals are unknowingly sprayed on our foods. This has a direct, consistent and significant impact on your thyroid health. These pesticides, insecticides, fungicides and other biocides stick to your thyroid gland like glue. They affect it badly. You must find a way to avoid foods that are not grown organically, or pay the extra premium for organic foods. There are so many studies. In 2010, scientists published an article that examined the association between using organochlorine insecticides and thyroid disease among women. After adjusting odds and getting their facts straight, the authors concluded there was an increased risk of hypothyroidism in women who were exposed. See page 99 to find out what medications you might be taking that have a chlorine backbone.

Question #5: What Kind of Water Do You Drink?

This is tough because drinking tap water gives you chlorine and fluorine. Drink from glass bottles as often as you can, the plastic water bottles are usually bad for your thyroid! It contains all sorts of chemicals. Plastics contain phthalates or bisphenol a (BPA), which majorly impacts thyroid signaling. Scientists evaluated various thyroid levels as well as urinary break down products (metabolites) of phthalate and BPA. The results were shocking. Among adults, there were significant inverse relationships between urinary metabolites of these toxins, and the amount produced of total T4, Free T4, total T3, and thyroglobulin; they also looked at TSH levels. Simply put, the higher the concentration of these breakdown compounds which come from plastic, the less thyroid hormones produced and the higher your TSH (not a good thing because it means you need more active thyroid hormone). There are many studies to show the relationship between plasticizers and suppressed thyroid function. If you really want to wake up your thyroid, you should drink out of glass bottles so you can avoid drinking the endocrine disrupting compounds.

Question #6: Do You Ask if the Fish is Wild-Caught?

Don't be shy on this one. It's better if it's wild-caught for dozens of reasons, the most important of which is this: Most fish raised in tight commercial captivity tanks would not stay alive if they weren't given all sorts of chemicals to keep them alive. Then they are injected with colors to make them look pretty so you will buy them. This is not the case with all farm-raised fish, there are some excellent, caring farms but it's hard to tell at a restaurant. It's better to just ask if it's wild-caught. If it's not, I'd pass, or eat just occasionally.

Avoid these Foods

Nutrients play a crucial role in helping to control thyroid disease. Generally speaking, the following food categories should be minimized or avoided altogether if you are struggling with severe hypothyroidism:

- ✓ Gluten-containing foods
- ✓ Soy based foods
- ✓ Cruciferous vegetables
- ✓ Heavily refined "junk" food
- ✓ Refined salt (ie table salt)
- ✓ White flour, tainted with alloxan (damages pancreas)
- ✓ Cereals and whole grains
- ✓ Alcohol

Chapter 23

Solutions for Thyroid Symptoms

I love simple solutions so later in this chapter I'm going to offer you a quick summary. Right now, here are 10 reasons why you have thyroid symptoms:

1. You have a shortage of Free T3.
   It takes one blood test to find out but it's hardly ordered! You can take T3 drugs too, but they are not routinely prescribed.

2. You have a shortage of Free T4.
   The basic recipe to make T4 is with tyrosine and iodine supplements, it's rare when a physician tells you to buy these 2 supplements!

3. Your thyroid is inflamed which slows down production of T4.
   You can easily measure antibodies to see if your thyroid is 'on fire' and inflamed. Selenium helps, and also, a rarely prescribed inexpensive medication called "low dose naltrexone" can help before too much thyroid destruction occurs.

4. You have liver inflammation.
   This prevents conversion from T4 to T3, yet liver cleanses and supplements are hardly every suggested. There are many including artichoke extract, milk thistle and liposomal glutathione.

5. You have poor gut flora.
   Probiotics are inexpensive but powerful, they convert 20% of your T4 to active T3 and can take some of you from hypothyroidism to wellness. One simple supplement, yet rarely ever suggested.

6. You lack basic nutrition.
   Let's not underestimate the power of a high-quality multivitamin or medical food. You see, all the cells in your body require basic building blocks to carry out the metabolic instructions that thyroid hormone gives them. None of us eat the way we should and poor nutrition equals fatigue and weight gain.

7. Your thyroid hormone is outside the cell.
   Remember, thyroid hormone sitting in the bloodstream does you little good. You need it inside the cell.

8. Omega 3 fatty acid deficiencies.
   Take a high quality EPA/DHA supplement, but not more than 500mg per day. Too much depletes your GLA. When you take fish oils, an omega 3 fatty acid, you have to also supplement with GLA (an omega 6 fatty acid) because high doses of fish oils will cause drug mugging of GLA. For example, if you take 1,000 mg of fish oil (EPA and DHA totaled together), you need 500mg GLA at the same time. Evening primrose oil supplements can provide this GLA. This is important because

GLA deficiency can increase your tendency to form clots (bad). GLA is known to protect the heart, without adequate amounts, you could suffer cardiac consequences, and this was not even addressed. Read my article entitled "New JAMA Study Bakes Fish Oils Don't Believe It." This is available at www.SuzyCohen.com.

9. You have a selenium deficiency.
   This could cause more antibodies and poor thyroid conversion. Selenium supplements can help because they improve T3 activation and transport. Selenium can reduce antibodies against the thyroid gland. Estrogen-containing drugs such as birth control and hormone replacement are 'drug muggers' of selenium, so by taking those medications, you indirectly suppress your thyroid hormone. Knowing this valuable information allows you to supplement with selenium for pennies a day and protect yourself from more damage done by the medications you need.

10. You have a high heavy metal load.
    I'm not excited about you yanking out your mercury fillings; let's start with simple things like avoiding tuna and Swordfish meals from now on, and quit smoking which causes cadmium to build up. You can see a biological dentist if you are really concerned about your dental fillings. I'm not saying not to, but sometimes shaking those loose causes more harm than good, so for now, stick with simple avoidance of heavy metals.

Thyroid Symptoms

With low thyroid there are symptoms to juggle and obviously, optimizing thyroid function helps heal the underlying cause. Until you get to a happy place, it's nice to know about simple, natural solutions that address the symptoms. I'll share what I've learned about some symptoms that aren't really dangerous, but annoying just the same. Up first, dry skin.

Dry Skin

You already know that you need to keep your skin hydrated, and I have lots of suggestions to help you do just that. Hydration is one key to alleviating dry skin but it isn't enough. You can drink a gallon of water or more and still have dry skin (and dry heels). If you add marshmallow root to your water and make a daily infusion of this, it will go miles in hydrating your skin. The thicker the better. There's a YouTube video of me teaching you how to make marshmallow infusion. Please watch that because the marshmallow infused water is naturally amazing! I also suggest that you consider omega 3 fatty acids, like fish oil. You can take one daily. A non-fish option is Chia Seed oil, like "Chia Omega" by Essential Formula's, Inc. And then there's Bioastin astaxanthin by Nutrex Hawaii. These are my go-to supplements for hydration. Here's another trick, apply coconut oil to your skin or hair, and cook with it too! Careful not to eat too much it can cause diarrhea.

The only thing I ask is that you don't slather on lotions that have harmful endocrine disruptors, which are chemicals that hurt your thyroid and reproductive organs. You can visit EWG's Skin Deep website which allows you to search the database and find out exactly what's in your lotion, toothpaste, shampoo, face cream, make up, and so forth. Here's the website: *www.ewg.org/skindeep/*.

Your goal is to avoid anything containing parabens, phthalates, and harsh sulfates. There are dozens of clean companies that make chemical-free lotions. I may not have eczema, but I can certainly speak to this dry skin problem because I live in a desert region of the United States, so I'm constantly trying to keep my skin soft and moisturized, especially in the winter. Aloe also repairs natural collagen which is damaged in people with eczema due to the destructive enzymes released during inflammation. (You know those destructive enzymes as cytokines or what we call "soldiers" in my book. Aloe contains hyaluronic acid, which helps plump the skin.

Thyroid Healthy Tip

Sometimes you have to get a chest X ray, or dental X ray or another X ray where your thyroid is potentially exposed depending on what's being imaged. Your thyroid gland is extremely sensitive to radiation, so I'd ask to wear a special collar during the X ray. Some collars are made with lead, and some are lead-free. Wrap it around your neck during the X ray. Not all imaging centers have these available, so if you'd like to bring your own, purchase it at a medical supply shop or online. The key search term to find one is "thyroid shield" or "thyroid collar."

Hair Loss or Thinning

Thyroid related hair loss is best managed when you optimize your thyroid but in the meantime, you should test yourself for iron and the storage form called ferritin. When iron is low, your hair will tend to fall out easier. Never take iron supplements at the same time as thyroid medicine. A study once showed that the supplement L-lysine could help too, follow label directions. Progesterone hormone may be low, especially during the second half of your monthly cycle. This means there is higher estrogen compared to progesterone. Low progesterone (high estrogen) increases thyroid binding globulin (TBG) which binds up active thyroid hormone so you feel more hypothyroid. You want your TBG levels to be somewhere between 13 and 39 µg/ml. Oral contraceptives increase your TBG that's why you feel worse if you take those pills or patches/shots. Some of you may benefit from progesterone medication or creams. I'd prefer that you get a bio-identical form of hormones from your doctor rather than buying the cream at a health food store. Most women do better on the oral "micronized" progesterone pills, than the transdermal ones, however this is very individual. Transdermal is okay with me, so long as it's bio-identical. The herb saw palmetto is sometimes used in low dosages for women with hair loss, and it's better known as a prostate formula. Weird, I know but true. Taking horsetail herb or silica will also help with hair growth.

I'm not giving out dosages here because I don't know what's right for all of you. I think you should start with very low dosages and get your doctor's approval first. Everything I mention here has side effects, especially the progesterone. I just want you to have some options. You will get to a healthier state, and for now be kind to yourself. If you want one of those hair pieces they sell at salons and beauty stores, go get one, they clip in and in 5 seconds, you feel pretty again.

Thinning Eyebrows

This is a very common sign of low thyroid, where the outer third (the edge) of your eyebrows thins or disappears. The same tips I suggested above for hair loss may help. In the meantime, an eyebrow pencil will work just fine. There's a neat little product called Renew Eyebrow Oil Formulation that could people have mentioned to me. It contains vitamins and herbs that could speed eyebrow regrowth. Ideally, you would restore thyroid hormone using medication or supplements, and your hair can grow back.

Dry Cracked Heels

Your heels get itchy due to the dryness and the skin starts to flake or crack when it gets real bad. Luckily, I have not yet experienced that, but they do get dry. I'm obsessed about keeping my heels moisturized. I love Skin Food moisturizer for this. You can also try this tonight. Gently scrub your feet with a pumice stone to remove dead skin cells. While still slightly wet, apply some TheraNeem Cream and then put on some old socks and go to sleep. You can do the same thing for your hands, just buy soft fabric gloves. The neem cream has all kinds of antioxidants and it feels very soothing.

Brain Fog & Depression

By far, this is the hardest symptom to address in people with low thyroid. If it's really low thyroid, then optimizing your levels of T4 and T3 will usually correct it. But sometimes people with hypothyroidism have brain fog for other reasons and therein lies the problem. If you optimize thyroid hormone, and the brain fog does not lift, that tells you it's related to something else. Maybe you have an infection like Lyme disease? This can cause brain fog. Maybe you have low levels of a brain hormone such as acetyl-choline which can lead to fuzzy thinking and poor memory. What if you got floxed from a fluoroquinolone antibiotic? If you don't know, refer to page 187. Adrenal fatigue can cause brain fog. There are so many causes for this, and just as many treatments. Some people say that molybdenum helps (about 50 to 100 mg, low doses) each day because it clears the acetylaldehyde out. My go to supplements for clear thinking include Acetyl L-carnitine, vinpocetine (about 10 twice daily but be careful it's a blood thinner), and siberian ginseng. If those don't help after a few months, con-sider bacopa and citicoline. Follow label directions or practitioner instructions.

I sometimes recommend neurotransmitter testing for people who feel depressed or anxious, even though testing is not 100% reliable. Your serotonin is made in your gut, dopamine in your kidneys, and other hormones in your brain. So the question remains where to measure a particular hormone. Urine and blood tests do not match if you take them simultaneously, plus, these tests do not always correlate with your clinical symptoms. I'm including them here because some doctors rely on them so I want you to know their limitations.

Are you prone to depression in the fall or spring? During the autumn and spring it can be 20 - 30 degrees colder or warmer from one day than the next, but it takes about a week for your thyroid gland to adjust to fluctuations in ambient temperatures. The constant ups and downs can overburden the thyroid system, making these seasons a potential disaster for some individuals. When I say disaster, I mean it, such as one complication called myxedema coma. Just knowing this fact allows you to protect yourself, and head it off with natural supplements that act as adaptogens and keep the signals to and from your thyroid flowing smoothly. These include ashwaghanda, rhodiola and schizandra. Remedies to help are sold at health food stores nationwide.

Right now, let's look how weird you can feel inside your mind when your neurotransmitters are imbalanced:

Dopamine. Deficiencies make you crave alcohol, illicit drugs, opiate painkillers and cigarettes. Correcting dopamine levels may help with addiction. But too much dopamine is associated with aggression and paranoia. Imbalances with this neurotransmitter (especially when low) are tied to Parkinson's, depression, attention/ focus problems, schizophrenia, spectrum disorders and autism.

Histamine. It makes you sneeze, but did you know that chronically high levels are tied to migraines, eczema and obsessive compulsive behavior? Low levels may cause chronic fatigue, low libido and paranoia.

Serotonin. Popular antidepressants lift it temporarily, including Celexa, Paxil and Zoloft. Deficiencies may cause fatigue, muscle cramps, irritability and a feeling of always being hot. High serotonin is tied to bone loss, irritable bowels, trembling and nausea.

If you're lacking norepinephrine, you may have profound adrenal fatigue and stubborn weight gain. If you're GABA-deficient, then insomnia and anxiety are evident to those around you. High epinephrine may make you too aggressive. Despite commercial ads, there isn't one pill to fix this. You have to undergo different tests, then use specific nutrients that push the correct metabolic pathway to produce the neurotransmitter or hormone you want.

Chronic Fatigue

The B vitamins are known to fight stress and fatigue so a simple option is B Complex. I'd like you to make sure that your brand contains only active, methylated B vitamins to make sure you absorb them. For example, your label should contain methylcobalamin for B12, not cyanocobalamin. And it should be "methylfolate" *not* folic acid. If you are taking folic acid, I would recommend switching to another brand that contains folinic acid, or 5-MTHF or quatrefolic, methylfolate.. These are active forms of B vitamins and it means you can use them, they are body-ready. Another example is "Pyridoxal 5' phosphate" not B6. If you don't buy a high-quality brand of B complex, you'll never get the full effects it could offer. If you have headaches, or severe fatigue, you want your supplement to contain "Riboflavin 5 phosphate" not plain riboflavin. Riboflavin is huge for people with methylation problems, high blood pressure and low thyroid. If you eat the Paleo diet, you're low in riboflavin. If you have low thyroid and methylation problems, it's double trouble and you should be taking extra riboflavin, or better yet, an active form riboflavin 5' phosphate.

I don't have confidence that your body can fully activate B vitamins found in plain regular B complex supplements, that's why I offer a supplement that contains all this for you, see my website *www.ScriptEssentials.com* (look for the B complex). Now, after a good B complex, I would recommend vitamin C because it improves happy brain chemicals and it encourages the production of neurotransmitters responsible for energy and joy. I'd also recommend adrenal nourishing adaptogens to help support cortisol balance. I would drink Tulsi tea all day long, any flavor. I would enhance intake of probiotics (Dr. Ohhira's Probiotics) because your gut microbiome is responsible for converting 20% of your thyroid hormone into T3 which makes a big difference in energy levels. There's a specialty product that I like called ATP Fuel and another called Energy Multi Plex, both by Researched Nutritionals. Those are fantastic and you can try one or both, and experiment. It's fine to include the other supplements I mention here along with those. For a quick boost, you can do drink one of the next 3 options:

1. Beet root shots, like "Red Ace" (by Brandstorm) it's so awesome!
2. Smoothie with almond milk and 1 scoop of rice or egg protein.
3. Yerba Mate shot by Guayaki, lime tangerine is my favorite.

Feeling Cold?

Buy a microwaveable hot pack. These bring pure joy in 60 seconds flat, which is all you need to heat it up in the microwave. I used to heat one up and tuck into bed at night with it. Sometimes, I just put it on my feet and it made me fall asleep faster and more comfy. What about the car? Do you dislike sitting on bone-chilling seats in your freezing car? If you're cold all the time, get a heated seat warmer. Plug it in your cigarette lighter and in a few minutes, your car seats are comfy. You can go to a salon and get a hot wax treatment for your hands, or your feet. This feels amazing!!! As for supplements, non-flush niacin will warm you up! You can try 100mg or 200mg that should do it. If not, you can go up to 500mg one time and the flushing should start within 15 to 30 minutes. I am not advising you to do this every day because you probably don't need niacin on a daily basis. I recommend it because it can help in times of 'emergency' like when your temperature drops to 94.5 or 95 and you are just freezing. This used to happen to Sam my husband so the 200 - 500 mg of plain niacin was a nice little 'rescue' remedy for him. You need to ask your doctor if this is okay for you. Cayenne pepper liquid herbal extract is another way to 'warm up' with a supplement, but it could burn your throat going down. Cayenne is known to support cardiovascular health. Herb Pharm makes a great brand.

Chapter 24

Live Thyroid Healthy

L et's get you well now! This final chapter is designed to offer you the "Script" I promised at the outset of my book, to help you get you well.

See a good doctor
Convert T4 to T3
Restore mugged nutrients
Interpret tests correctly
Protect your thyroid gland from casein/gluten/soy
Transport thyroid hormone into your cells

As you've learned, in order to live thyroid healthy, you need to give your body T3 and that is what provides energy, burns fat, clears cobwebs from your brain and warms you up. Nourishing adrenal glands is important. No one with thyroid disease has healthy adrenals, I assure you. These go hand in hand, no matter what you are told. Sometimes you have to literally discontinue your thyroid medication, take some adrenal adaptogens, or some hydrocortisone medication for a week or two, and then restart your thyroid medication. You will have to start secreting a more active form of TSH, and you will have to have your transport system working well, remember most of the conversion of T4 to T3 (compliments of those "D" enzymes) happens inside your cells. To get the T4 into the cell, you have to make those receptors sticky, like glue. This is referred to as receptor binding. When you have problems in any of these areas, it is referred to by conventional medicine as "secondary" or "tertiary" hypothyroidism, and they say it's "rare." And let me tell you this kind of thinking is exactly the kind of thinking that keeps you thyroid sick! In my book, it is common, and huge, and knowing it's happening to you is the answer to your prayers. If someone tells you that secondary hypothyroidism is rare, they don't know what they're talking about.

I suspect that, like many people who have heard me speak about this at lectures and book signings, you are probably mad. I get dozens of people come up to me after lectures and say how mad they are at their doctors, for not having been told this after paying thousands of dollars for lab tests, medicines, scans and imaging, special diets and so on (lost days at work for feeling so badly, or having migraines). I hear ya! But that's what you have me for, and that's why it's so important to my work, if you learn something that helps you to please leave me a 5 star review on Amazon. I really need those, please tell others about me. Can you imagine what I'm up against here, as a pharmacist? Most pharmacists quietly dispense the medication day in, day out, by the thousands each week.

And all I want to do is help you feel better... make your days better, help you lose weight, look beautiful, relieve pain and sleep easier. You know I'm going to get a lot of lip from people who don't know this information and refuse to read the references I've provided in the back of my book. Sigh.

On a good note, being that I'm a practitioner for the Institute of Functional Medicine, I am friends with and respected by many practitioners from different avenues. Practitioners from all over the world they rely on me to help shine a light into dark corners of research, I make their job easier by educating you, and empowering you ... and then you find your way to these wonderful practitioners. But you're reading my book right now, and I'm here to help get the ball rolling, so you can finally become thyroid healthy, just like I promised at the outset of this book. Here's my suggested S-C-R-I-P-T to help you get well:

See a good doctor
Convert T4 to T3
Restore mugged nutrients
Interpret tests correctly
Protect your thyroid gland from casein/gluten/soy
Transport thyroid hormone into your cells

S is for "See a Good Doctor"

This is Step 1

This is the first place to start if you want to become thyroid healthy. Have you not given your current treatment plan a few months, or a few years by now? If it isn't working, I suggest you educate your physician or find a different doctor who can give you back your life. You are paying them you know?! You can continue paying someone because you love him/her, or you can pay someone to give you vibrant health again (like them or not). For me, it's about the outcome, the incredible results, feeling happy and healthy, and sexy and strong... and less about their personality or office staff. Ask at a compound pharmacy if they know someone who specializes in thyroid health. To find a local compounding pharmacy in your area, you can use this site: *www.ecompoundingpharmacy.com*.

Don't be afraid to call around to local doctor's offices. Ask the staff (before you pay to see them) how they test their patients, and ask specifically if they base their treatments on the TSH and T4 test? Ask if they ever measure Reverse T3 or antibodies as a general rule. You can also find your dream doctor by going to functionalmedicine.org and putting in your zip code, this will pull up physicians that understand what I've been saying in my book. Also, naturopaths can speak this language and help you in ways that conventional physicians cannot since they use more natural approaches, I've included a link for their site below, along with other sites to help you locate your dream doctor. I can't be responsible if one of these turns out to be a nightmare, as opposed to your dream doctor. I'm just trying to help, in alphabetical order:

American Association of Naturopathic Physicians:
  http://www.naturopathic.org/AF_MemberDirectory.asp?version=1
American Board of Integrative Holistic Medicine, Physician
  Locator: *http://www.abihm.org/search-doctors*
Functional Medicine (I am a practitioner of this type of
  medicine, and all my other health books are based on their
  principles). Love this site! *http://www.functionalmedicine.org/*
  practitioner_search.aspx?id=117#results
Thyroid Change site. This is an excellent site on many levels,
  and this particular page can help you find a doctor in the
  United States, Australia and Canada.
  http://www.thyroidchange.org/list-of-doctors.html
Thyroid UK site. They have a link for their own physicians,
  local to you if you live there: *http://www.thyroiduk.org.uk/*
  tuk/diagnosis/private_doctors.html
Top Thyroid Doctors Directory: *http://www.thyroid-*
  info.com/topdrs/index.htm
Thyroid Doctors: Sponsored by RLC Labs, producer of Nature-
  throid and WP Thyroid (formerly Westhroid Pure). Locate a
  doctor: *http://thyroiddoctors.com*
Paleo Physicians Network. This is a great site that offers more
  information about the Paelo diet which I highly recommend
  for most people (not all) but definitely people with autoimmune disorders. They can help you find a natural-minded
  doctor who is familiar with the Paleo diet in the United States,
  Germany, New Zealand, Canada, France, Finland and more:
  http://paleophysiciansnetwork.com/ (Not all the doctors listed
  there are experts specifically in thyroid disease.)

C is for "Convert T4 to T3"

This is Step 2. It has to be done or you'll remain thyroid sick. There's no way you're getting around this part. If that conversion takes place, you have more T3 and it's your biologically active 'wake-me-up' thyroid hormone. There are specific minerals and nutrients that are needed to improve activation, there are adaptogenic herbs like ashwagandha that improve this conversion.

Nutrient Depletions	Stress	Aging	Alcohol	Obesity
Chemo-therapy	Cigarettes	Diabetes	Fasting	Soy
Medications	Goitrogens	Pesticides	Radiation	Surgery
Kidney & Liver disease	Heavy Metals	Growth Hormone Deficiency	Low Progesterone	Iodine Excess

Dr. David Brownstein "Overcoming Thyroid Disorders"
www.DrBrownstein.com

R is for "Restore Mugged Nutrients"

This is Step 3. You have to put back what's missing: You are being robbed of nutrients from your food, refined sugar, coffee, wine and medicines. We know that medications wipe out our probiotics, and that reduces conversion of 20% of thyroid hormone, so replenishing beneficial bacteria is important to your thyroid, not to mention your gastrointestinal tract! Beyond probiotics, there are hundreds of thousands of medications that are drug muggers of your nutrients. When you take a drug that reduces your minerals and B vitamins, you can no longer make thyroid hormone, nor can you convert it to its active form. You will become thyroid sick until you restore those "mugged" nutrients. You should refer to Chapter 7,

Restore Mugged Nutrients to learn about specific thyroid thieves. You should also a copy off Amazon of my *Drug Muggers* book which gives you a book full of information to do this properly as well as dietary choices to restore lost nutrients. There's an art, you don't just take this pill or that one, you have to time nutrients away from your thyroid medicine, you also have to buy high-quality vitamins or you'll just make expensive urine.

Finally, if you've been drinking coffee, soda or energy shots to get you through your day, I want to tell you those are 'drug muggers' of minerals, the minerals you need to make and convert thyroid hormone. Restoring mugged nutrients can breathe life into you very quickly.

I is for "Interpret Tests Correctly"

This is Step 4. You need to learn a little more about how to read your lab tests and interpret them. For example, you need to know that when your physician says "Look, your TSH is within normal limits because it is 3" that this is an incorrect interpretation, one that leaves you feeling bad.

I've spent a great deal of time in this book teaching you how to get properly tested, and how to interpret your results so that you can get yourself well. The reason is because you have been banging your head for years, quietly resigning yourself to the fact that your thyroid tests are "normal" with the black and white results in front of you prove it. You have been laying out hard earned cash for your doctor and pharmacy taking drugs you don't need (pain killers, antidepressants, stimulants, fibromyalgia drugs) and all you really need is thyroid hormone! No more baby! I want you to get an attitude now, muster it up, and fight for adequate testing. Thyroid is my bitch! That is your new motto, and you will demand that your lab tests be done correctly, and interpreted properly or you'll get a new doctor. Well documented studies prove TSH test doesn't work well. Correct interpretation makes or breaks you!

P is for "Protect Your Thyroid Gland

This is Step 5. It is all about protection. I'd recommend you eat a very clean diet, one that consists of organic fruits and vegetables, nuts and seeds and 'clean' meats. What I mean by clean is grass-fed, hormone free lean proteins. I'd love to see you juice frequently, and take protein shots such as rice, pea or hemp protein supplements in your smoothie. The biggest deal though, bigger than anything is the avoidance of food antigens that hurt your thyroid gland. Casein from dairy and gluten from wheat based foods are top of the list, and of course soy because it is a goitrogen (it lowers thyroid production), plus it is usually GMO. If you don't want to avoid gluten and dairy, at the very least consider a digestive enzyme such as DPPIV to help reduce absorption in your gut. This is discussed in Chapter 21, *Foods That Can Keep You Thyroid Sick*. I've included DPPIV in ThyroScript capsules (*www.Script Essentials.com*) which I formulated to support thyroid health. The unique combination contains essential vitamins and minerals to improve conversion of T4 into T3, it's anti-fungal, plus it has the digestive enzyme to protect your thyroid gland from casein and gluten.

T is for "Transport Thyroid Hormone into Your Cells"

Step 6. No matter how much thyroid hormone you make, it has to get inside your cells (tissues). It doesn't do any good sitting in your blood stream, you need it to get INSIDE the cell. Your body has an active transport system so it's shuttled in, it doesn't just passively flow in. This is old school thinking. You can support the transport mechanism by eating nutrient dense foods and taking nutrients and supplements which improve cell membrane integrity like sunflower lecithin which offers a form of soy-free phosphatidylcholine. Did you know that every cell in your body needs cholesterol for the cell membrane? It helps with the transport system. If you reduce your cholesterol too much, you get unhealthy cell membranes. By the way, heart disease isn't caused by high cholesterol, it's caused by inflammation in the arteries. If you run out of vitamin C you can't make collagen, and then your body lays down cholesterol and plaque in the arteries to patch up the tiny little cracks. Heart attacks are not caused by a statin deficiency (wink wink). Vitamin C is important to keeping your arteries flexible and intact, and I think it's more helpful than medication which reduces your production of cholesterol (never sweeping clean your arteries). As for cell membranes, I also like astaxanthin (BioAstin by Nutrex Hawaii) because it is a protective antioxidant that protects the inner and outer part of our cells, and cell membrane.

A naturopathic doctor, or nutritionist may have some opinions about what nutrients, and what special formulas are specifically helpful for you. Right now, I'd like to focus on some of the best nutrients and herbs that could support healthy thyroid function and do all of the things I just said were important. The nutrients and herbs I'm about to discuss are all available at health food stores and herbal apothecaries. You can buy each of them and try it on it's own, but do not add any more than 1 supplement at full dose, per week in case you react. If you were to develop some kind of side effect, for example diarrhea, then you would have trouble sorting out which supplement it was if you go to fast and add several new supplements in one day. I know I know, you are anxious to get well fast but going slowly is better for you. Buying all of the supplements below could get expensive so maybe just try two or three of them.

As an option, I have my own formula called ThyroScript which is a blend of key nutrients which improve T3 conversion and anti-inflammatory herbs and adaptogens. I'm very proud of this, it has been several years in the making and it's available now. I've based my formula upon my years of research into this area, and personal experience with low thyroid. The combination of ingredients is very gentle and offers synergy. It may or may not be fine to take with your thyroid medicine. Like most thyroid supplements, they enhance the effect of thyroid drugs which could be good or bad depending on many individual factors. More information on ThyroScript is available at *www.ScriptEssentials.com* where I have a "FAQ" tab for frequently asked questions. Before taking supplement, ask a holistic minded practitioner before beginning.

Thyroid Make-Over

Now that you've read my "Script" to get thyroid healthy, I want to talk about other changes you make. You have so much power in this situation, and I want your healing to take place as fast as possible. It's basically a thyroid make-over!

What Else Can You Do?

+ Include protein with every meal. You can either eat it (as in meat, seafood or eggs), or you can take a protein shake each morning. Even if you are vegan, you can do this because there are proteins made with pea, rice or hemp today. It's not all whey and egg like it used to be.

+ Reduce carbohydrates. If you can go grain free (or Paleo) I'm even happier. Did you know studies prove that reducing your intake of high-glycemic index carbohydrate (such as refined grain products) could help you from overeating? Highly processed, refined junk food or simple carbohydrates stimulate brain regions and cause cravings. The blood sugar swings are bad for you.

+ Reduce or eliminate caffeine. This may be something you need right now but if you can reduce it I think you'll feel better. If feel like you need the stimulating effect, lean into the process by drinking yerba mate shots or teas, Runa's guayusa tea or Tulsi tea which all offer a nice lift. Juice carrots with kale or Swiss chard, along with an apple and small piece of turmeric. It will give you a good lift too.

✦ Relax. Get a massage or ask your partner to trade 15 minutes with you, each getting a little massage. If that doesn't work, just lay in the dark with a glowing lamp and soft soundscape music playing. Take a hot bath ... anything, the goal here is to turn off the stress for a few minutes. Your thyroid and adrenals need to catch a break sometimes.

✦ Correct adrenal glands problems. I'm very compassionate about this, and recognize we are all under stress of some sort. As I take off in a plane, I'm aware that each 'box' down there (house) has a story, everyone is struggling with some issue, or health concern. If they aren't, someone they love is. Suffering is universal, we each experience it a different way. You may not have suffered anything major in your life in terms of 'the human struggle' like I have, but even the microstressors in the background of your life take a toll. Chronic stress reduces the cell's ability to absorb thyroid hormone by 50-79%. The more stress you are under, the worse your thyroid function will be. It's the never-ending email, deadlines at work, the exes, the to-do list, the laundry pile up on the couch, that book you were supposed to return, the voice mails, the 'Thank You' cards you should write, the plane tickets you need to buy, the mileage log, snow to be shoveled, etcetera. Nothing's a big deal, but it adds up and weighs on you. It's not the same hit on your adrenals as a scare you might get when you swerve to avoid a dog in the road, no, it's actually much worse because the pile of microstressors never ends. A hamster wheel of deadlines and obligations. This can tax your adrenals and I promise you, there's no faster way to fix your thyroid than to nurture your adrenals first. You have to lighten your responsibility load or health is at stake. Sometimes you have to discontinue your thyroid medication, take some hydrocortisone medication for a week or two, and then restart your thyroid medication. This is particularly effective for people who have low levels of adrenal hormones.

10 Reasons Why You're Not Feeling better

I'm going to do a little countdown now, starting with the 10th reason.

10 You're getting into gluten or GMO corn every day without knowing it. Many thyroid supplements use modified food starch that contains gluten or corn. Some of it's GMO'd and that can stimulate your cytokines and inflammation. It lights your thyroid on fire. In fact, you don't even have to be super sensitive, GMOs and gluten are additives and they can be harmful to anyone.

9 You're genes are playing tricks with you. If you have a genetic mutation such that you can't methylate well, then you're not making enough glutathione, a master antioxidant that cleans your body up. You may need extra folate to clear the toxins. You can test for genetic issues with 23andMe testing, it requires a saliva sample. *www.23andMe.com*. Opening up blocked pathways in your body can make a huge difference, and it may also require certain dietary restrictions, low sulfur foods and supplements.

8 You're eating thyroid-killing foods and chemicals that contain fluorine, bromine or chlorine. Read Chapter 8, *Thyroid Thieves Lurking Everywhere.*

7 You haven't reduced antibodies and put that thyroid fire
   out, while igniting your adrenals to work better. Track
   your thyroid antibodies and make sure they're normal
   because sometimes those will be sky high even with
   normal perfect TSH and T4.

6 You're not detoxifying properly. Perhaps you have
   constipation? This means you are not 'taking out the
   garbage.' Perhaps you are dehydrated? Then all your
   poisons are concentrated in your bloodstream. Your
   kidneys have to deal with that. Maybe you have liver
   dysfunction?

5 You're eating foods that look like gluten to your body.
   Cross-reactivity is a big problem, that's why I tell most
   people to eat a grain free diet. Some of you know you're
   allergic to gluten, and you stay away from it, but other
   grains (rice, corn, amaranth, spelt, quinoa) act the same
   way in your body and cause your thyroid to be on fire.
   Casein, the protein from dairy (a biggie!) and coffee
   particles also look like gluten to an inflamed thyroid
   gland. It's because cross-reactive foods have proteins
   which look similar to gluten and thus, trigger the same
   immune response as if you were eating gluten.

4 You're eating cereal and snack bars for breakfast. Not
   only do these contain grains which I recommend you
   avoid, they also do nothing to help you balance blood
   sugar. Eat a breakfast with protein and fresh, organic
   fruits and vegetables. At the very least, juice several time
   a week. Use vitamin A loaded items and also those with
   minerals. I like to put in cantaloupe with carrots, an
   orange, some lettuce leaves, and a leaf of kale. You can

also try a smoothie instead, made with hemp protein and almond milk.

3 You're deficient in minerals. If you drink coffee, it's safe to assume you are deficient, and this means you won't have enough selenium, magnesium, zinc, iron and other trace minerals to activate your thyroid hormone. Magnesium is important because it is essential for the production for ATP formation. You will need a good trace mineral supplement if you drink coffee because it steals magnesium and iron, don't forget that. If you take a trace mineral supplement, take it away from your thyroid medicine. Minerals activate your T3 hormone and help you with the transport systems to put that thyroid hormone into your cell (where you want it).

2 You're thyroid medicine is incorrect. There are many options and having the right medicine for you can breathe life into you within days. It is just amazing to me how everyone reacts differently to each medicine. I wish I could tell you which drug worked best but we are all unique. I just know that when you get this part right, you feel better.

1 You have adrenal fatigue! If you don't nourish your adrenal glands for a few weeks or months then you won't respond to your thyroid medicine. If you've been under any kind of stress, chances are good that your pilot light has petered out and you won't respond to thyroid. Pump in higher and higher doses of thyroid and it won't matter. This is the #1 cause for people to not respond to thyroid medicine in my book. Adrenals matter the most. There is an entire chapter in my

Headache Free book if you'd like to read about the connection to migraines and menstrual headaches.

Searching for More Information on Thyroid Illness?

There are many books on the topic, however most of them just rehash the same old news. If you would like fresh perspective, and more details, refer to some of the books in my personal library. These are some excellent resources, written by my good friends in this field. I've listed them in alphabetical order and each has their own special focus as it pertains to thyroid disease:

David Brownstein, MD is a physician in Michigan specializing in complex diseases using integrative Functional Medicine approaches. He's written 12 national best-sellers including *Overcoming Thyroid Disorders.* He also wrote the book on *Iodine: Why You Need it, Why You Can't Live Without It.* He is a great doctor, and friend. Free newsletter is available at his website, *www.DrBrownstein.com*

Alan Christianson, MD is a doctor in the Phoenix area specializing in Functional Medicine, hormone balancing and thyroid disease. He wrote *The Complete Idiot's Guide to Thyroid Disease. www.IntegrativeHealthcare.com*

Gena Lee Nolin, former Baywatch beauty and thyroid thriver, wrote in tandem with Mary J. Shomon, the best-seller, *Beautiful Inside and Out, Conquering Thyroid Disease With a Healthy, Happy, "Thyroid Sexy" Life. www.officialgenaleenolin.com*

Mary J. Shomon, a popular thyroid advocate on About.com which has fabulous articles wrote *Living Well With Hypothyroidism What Your Doctor Doesn't Tell You ... That You Need to Know.* She also wrote *Living Well With Graves' and Hyperthyroidism. www.thyroid.about.com*

Izabella Wentz, Pharm D and Marta Nowosadzka, MD. This mom and daughter dynamo will teach you everything you need to know to get well if you have Hashimoto's disease and complications. Even if you have had the condition for years, you will find many tips to regain your health. *Hashimoto's Thyroiditis: Lifestyle Interventions for Finding and Treating the Root Cause. www.ThyroidPharmacist.com* for free newsletter and articles.

References

Ahima RS, et al. Role of leptin in the neuroendocrine response to fasting. *Nature* 382: 1996; 250-252.

Akçay M, Akçay G. The presence of the antigliadin antibodies in autoimmune thyroid diseases. *Hepatogastroenterology*. 2003 Dec;50 Suppl 2:cclxxix-cclxxx.

Altomonte L et al. Serum levels of interleukin-1alpha, tumor necrosis factor-alpha and interleukin-2 in rheumatoid arthritis. Correlation with disease activity. *Clin. Rheumatol* 1992;11(2)202–205.

Andra G et al. Serum leptin in children with obesity. Relationship to gender and development. *Pediatrics* 1996;98:201-203.

Araujo RL, Andrade BM, da Silva ML, et al. Tissue-specific deiodinase regulation during food restriction and low replacement dose of leptin in rats. *Am J Physiol Endocinol Metab* 2009;296:E1157-E1163.

Arem R, Wiener GJ, Kaplan SG, Kim HS, et al. Reduced tissue thyroid hormone levels in fatal illness. *Metabolism* 1993;42(9):1102-8.

Baumgartner A, Graf KJ, Kurten I, Meinhold H. The hypothalamic-pituitary-thyroid axis in psychiatric patients and healthy subjects. *Psychiatry Research* 12988;24:271-332.

Beard J. et al. Impaired thermoregulation and thyroid function in iron-deficiency anemia. *Am J Clin Nutr.* 1990 Nov; 52(5): 813-9.

Benker G, Raida M, Olbricht T. et al. TSH Secretion In Cushing's Syndrome: Relation To Glucocorticoid Excess, Diabetes, Goitre, And The 'Sick Euthyroid Syndrome'. *Clin Endocrinol* 1990;33(6):777-86.

Bianco AC, Nunes MT, Hell NS, Maciel RMB. The Role of Glucocorticoids in the Stress-Induced Reduction of Extrathyroidal 3,5,3 -Triiodothyronine Generation in Rats. *Endocrinology* 1987 120: 1033-1038.

Bianco AC, Salvatore D, Gereben B, Berry MJ, Larsen PR. Biochemistry, Cellular and Molecular Biology, and Physiological Roles of the Iodothyronine Selenodeiodinases. *Endocrine Reviews* 2002;23 (1):38-89.

Brabant G, Brabant A, Ranft U, Ocran K et al. Circadian and Pulsatile Thyrotropin Secretion in Euthyroid Man Under the Influence of Thyroid Hormone and Glucocorticoid Administration. *J Clin Endocrinol Metab* 1987; 65: 83-88.

Brent GA, Hershman JM. Thyroxine therapy in patients with severe nonthyroidal illnesses and low serum thyroxine concentration. *J Clin Endocrinol Metab* 1986;63(1):1-8.

Campos-Barros A, Hoell T, Musa A, Sampaolo S, et al. Phenolic and tyrosyl ring iodothyronine deiodination and thyroid hormone concentrations in the human central nervous system. *J Clin Endocrinol Metab* 1996; 81:2179–2185.

Cavalieri RR, Castle JN, McMahon FA. Effects of dexamethasone on kinetics and distribution of triiodothyronine in the rat. *Endocrinology* 1984;114:215–221.

Cettour-Rose P, Burger AG, Meier CA, Visser TJ, et al. Central stimulatory effect of leptin on T3 production is mediated by brown adipose tissue type II deiodinase. *Am J Physiology Endocrinol Metab* 2002;283(5): E980-7.

Chatenoud L et al. Whole grain food intake and cancer risk. *Int J Cancer.* 1998 Jul 3;77(1):24-8.

Cheron RG, Kaplan MM, Larsen PR. Physiological and pharmacological influences on thyroxine to 3,5,3'-triiodothyronine conversion and nuclear 3,5,3'-triiodthyroidne binding in rat anterior pituitary. *J Clin Invest* 1979;64:1402-1414.

Chopra IJ, Chopra U, Smith SR, et al. Reciprocal changes in serum concentrations of 3,3',5-triiodothyronine (T3) in systemic illnesses. *J Clin Endocrinol Metab* 1975;41:1043–9.

Chopra IJ, Williams DE, Orgiazzi J, Solomon DH. Opposite effects of dexamethasone on serum concentrations of 3,3_,5_- triiodothyronine (reverse T3) and 3,3_,5-triiodothyronine (T3). *J Clin Endocrinol Metab* 1975;41:911–920.

Chopra IJ. A study of extrathyroidal conversion of thyroxine (T4) to 3,3',5-triiodothyronine (T3) in vitro. *Endocrinology.* 1977 Aug;101(2):453-63.

Clausen P, Mersebach H, Nielsen B, et al. Hypothyroidism is associated with signs of endothelial dysfunction despite 1-year replacement therapy with levothyroxine. *Clinical Endocrinology* 2009;70:932–937.

Cole DP, Thase ME, Mallinger AG, et al. Slower treatment response in biolar depression predicted by lower pretreatment thyroid function. *Am J Psychiatry* 2002; 159:116–121.

Considine RV, Sinha MK, Heiman ML, Kriauciunas A, et al. Serum immunoreactive-leptin. concentrations in normal-weight and obese humans *New England Journal Medicine* 1996;334: 292-295.

Cooper DS, Biondi B. Subclinical thyroid disease. *Lancet.* 2012 Mar 24;379(9821):1142-54.

Croxson MS, Ibbertson HK, Low serum triiodothyronine (T3) and hypothyroidism in anorexia nervosa. *J Clin Endorinol Metab* 1977;44:167-174.

Croxson MS, Ibbertson HK. Low serum triiodothyronine (T3) and hypothyroidism. *J clin Endocrinol Metab* 1977;44:167-174.

Dagogo_Jack S. Human Leptin Regualtion and Promis in Pharmacotheroapy. *Current Drug Targets* 2001;2:181-195.

Dagogo-Jack S, Tanellis C, Paramore D, Diother 3J, Land TM. Plasma Leptin and Insulin Relationships in Obese and Nonobese Human, *Diabetes* 1996;45:695-698.

De Groot Leslie J, Non-Thyrodial illness syndrome is a manifestation of hypothalamic-pituitary dysfunction, and in view of current evidence, should be treated with appropriate replacement therapies. *Crit Care Clin* 2006;22:57-86.

De Jong M. Docter R, van der Hoek HJ, Vos RA. Transport of 3,5,3'-tri-iodothyronine into the perfused rat liver and subsequent metabolism are inhibited by fasting. *Endocrinology* 1992;131(1):463-470.

De Marinis L, Mancini A, Masala R, et al. Evaluation of pituitary-thyroid axis response to acute myocardial infarction. *J Endocrinol Invest* 1985;8:507–11.

DeGroot LJ. Non-thyroidal illness syndrome is functional central hypothyroidism, and if severe, hormone replacement is appropriate in light of present knowledge. *J Endocrinol Invest* 2003;26:1163-1170.

Diane T. Thyroid-stimulating autoantibodies may yield relevant biomarkers for pediatric Graves' disease. *J Clin Endocrinol Metab.* 2014; doi:10.1210/jc.2013-4026.

Doyle D. Benzodiazepines inhibit temperature dependent L-[125I] triiodothyronine accumulation into human liver, human neuroblast, and rat pituitary cell lines. *Endocrinology* 1992;130:1211-1216.

Drutel A, Archambeaud F, Caron P. Selenium and the thyroid gland: more good news for clinicians. *Clin Endocrinol (Oxf).* 2013 Feb;78(2):155-64.

du Pont JS. Is reverse T3 a physiological nonactive competitor of the action of T3 upon the electrical properties of GH3 cells? *Neuroendo* 1991;54:146-150.

Duick DS, Warren DW, Nicoloff JT, Otis CL, Croxson MS. Effect of single dose dexamethasone on the concentration of serum triiodothyronine in man. *J Clin Endocrinol Metab* 1974;39:1151-1154.

Duntas LH. Resveratrol and its impact on aging and thyroid function. Endocrinol Invest. 2011 Nov;34(10):788-92.

Duval F, Mokrani MC, Bailey P, Correa H, et al. Thyroid axis activity and serotonin function major depressive episode. *Psychoneuroendocrinology* 1999;24:695-712.

Effects of obesity, total fasting and re-alimentation on L-thyroxine (T 4), 3,5,3-L-triiodothyronine (T3), 3,3,5-L-triiodothyronine (rT3), thyroxine binding globulin (TBG), transferrin, 2 –haptoglobin and complement C3 in serum. *Acta Endocrinol* 1979;91:629–43.

Ellingsen DG, Efskind J, Haug E, Thomassen Y, Martinsen I, Gaarder PI. Effects of low mercury vapour exposure on the thyroid function in chloralkali workers. *J Appl Toxicol*.2000;20(6):483-9.

Elliot DL, Goldberg L, Kuehl KD, Bennett WM. Sustained depression of the resting metabolic rate after massive weight loss. *Am J Clin Nutr* 1989;49:93-6.

Enia G, et al. Subclinical hypothyroidism is linked to micro-inflammation and predicts death in continuous ambulatory peritoneal dialysis. *Nephrol Dial Transplant*. 2007 Feb;22(2):538-44. Epub 2006 Nov 2.

Escobar-Morreale HF, Escobar del Rey F, Obregon MJ, Morreale de Escobar G. Only the combined treatment with thyroxine and triiodothryoidine ensures euthyroidism in all tissue… *Endocrinology* 1996;137:2490-2502.

Escobar-Morreale HF, Obregon MJ, Escobar del Rey F, Morreale de Escobar G. Replacement therapy for hypothyroidism with thyroxine alone does not ensure euthyroidism in all tissue. *J Clin Invest* 1995;96(6):2828–2838.

Everts ME, Lim C-F, Moerings EPCM, Docter R, et al. Effects of a furan fatty acid and indoxyl sulfate on thyroid hormone uptake in cultured anterior pituitary cells. *Am J Physiol* 1995;268:E974-E979.

Everts ME, Visser TJ, Moerings EM, Docter R, et al. Uptake of triiodothyroacetic acid and its effect on thyrotropin secretion in cultered anterior pituitary cells. *Endocrinology* 1994;135(6):2700-2707.

Fekete C et al. Differential Effects of Central Leptin, Insulin, or Glucose Administration during Fasting on the Hypothalamic-Pituitary-

Thyroid Axis and Feeding-Related Neurons in the Arcuate Nucleus. *Endocrinology* 2006;147(1):520-529.

Fontana L, Klein S, Holloszy JO, Premachandra BN. Effect of long-term calorie restriction with adequate protein and micronutrients on thyroid hormones. *J Clin Endocrinol Metab* 2006;91(8):3232-3235.

Forhead AJ, Curtis K, Kaptein E, Visser TJ, Fowden Al. Developmental Control of Iodothyronine Deiodinases by Cortisol in the Ovine Fetus and Placenta Near Term. *Endocrinology* 2006;147:5988-5994

Forman-Hoffman V, Philibert RA. Lower TSH and higher T4 levels are associated with current depressive syndrome in young adults. *Acta Psychiatry Scand* 2006;114:132-139.

Franceschi, S et al. Diet and thyroid cancer: a pooled analysis of four European case-control studies. *Int J Cancer.* 1991 May 30;48(3):395-8.

Francon J, Cantoux F, Blondeau JP. Carrier-mediated transport of thyroid hormones into rat glial cells in primary culture. *J Neurochem* 1989;53:1456–1463.

Friberg L, et al. Association between increased levels of reverse triiodothyronine and mortality after acute myocardial infarction *Am J Med.*2001;111(9):699-703.

Germain DL. Metabolic effect of 3,3 ,5 -triiodothyronine in cultured growth hormone-producing rat pituitary tumor cells. Evidence for a unique mechanism of thyroid hormone action. *J Clin Invest* 1985;76(2):890–893.

Girvent M, Maestro S, Hernandez R, et al. Euthyroid sick syndrome, associated endocrine abnormalities, and outcome in elderly patients undergoing emergency operation. *Surgery* 1998;123:560–7.

Gitlin M, Altshuler LL, Frye MA, Suri M, Huynh EL, et al. Peripheral thyroid hormones and response to selective serotonin reuptake inhibitors. *J Psychiatry Neurosci* 2004;29(5):383-386.

Giynas A, et al. The prevalence of depression and anxiety disorders in patients with euthyroid Hashimoto's thyroiditis: a comparative study. *Gen Hosp Psychiatry.* 2014 Jan-Feb; 36(1): 95-8.

Gold MS, Pottash LC, Extein I. Hypothyroidism and depression. *JAMA* 1981;245(19):1919-1922.

Goldner WS, et al. Pesticide use and thyroid disease among women in the Agricultural Health Study. *Am J Epidemiol.* 2010 Feb 15;171(4): 455-64.

Gomez C, Bandez MJ, Navarro A. Pesticides and impairment of mitochondrial function in relation with the Parkinsonian syndrome. *Front Biosci* 2007;12:1079–93.

Grossmann M, et al. Measuring thyroid peroxidase antibodies on the day nulliparous women present for management of miscarriage: a descriptive cohort study. *Reprod Biol Endocrinol.* 2013 May 14; 11-40.

Krenning EP, Docter R, Bernard HF, et al. The essential role of albumin in the active transport of thyroid hormones into primary cultured rat hepatocytes. *FEBS Lett* 1979;1;107(1):227-30.

Haddow JE, et al. Maternal thyroid deficiency during pregnancy and subsequent neuropsychological development of the child. *N Engl J Med.* 1999 Aug 19;341(8):549-55.

Hak AE, et al. Subclinical hypothyroidism is an independent risk factor for atherosclerosis and myocardial infarction in elderly women: the Rotterdam Study. *Ann Intern Med.* 2000 Feb 15;132(4):270-8.

Hashimoto H, Igarashi N, Yachie A, Miyawaki T, et al. The relationship between serum levels of interleukin-6 and thyroid hormone in children with acute respiratory infection. *J Clin Endocrinol* Metab 1994;78: 288-291.

Hatterer JA, Herbert J, Jidaka C, Roose SP, Gorman JM. CSF transthyretin in patients with depression *Am J Psychiatry* 1993;150:813-815.

Heimeier RB, Buchholz DR, Shi. YB. The xenoestrogen bisphenol A inhibits postembryonic vertebrate development by antagonizing gene regulation by thyroid hormone. *Endocrinology* 2009;150(6): 2964-2973.

Hennemann G, Docter R, Friesema EC, De Jong M, et al. Plasma membrane transport of thyroid hormones and its role in thyroid hormone metabolism and bioavailability. *Endocrine Reviews* 2001;22(4):451-476.

Hennemann G, Krenning EP, Bernard B, Huvers F, et al. Regulation of Influx and efflux of thyroid hormones in rat hepatocytes: Possible physiologic significance of plasma membrane in the regulation of thyroid hormone activity. *Horm Metab Res Suppl* 1984;14:1-6.

Hennemann G, Vos RA, de Jong M, et al. Decreased peripheral 3,5,3'-triiodothyronine (T3) production from thyroxine (T4): A syndrome of impaired thyroid hormone activation due to transport inhibition of T4- into T3-producing tissues. *J Clin Endocrinol Metabol* 1993;77(5):1431-1435.

Hennenmann G, Everts ME, de Jong M, et al. The significance of plasma membrane transport in the bioavailability of thyroid hormone. *Clin Endo* 1998;48:1-8.

Holtorf Kent. www.NAhypothyroidism.org

Iglesias P, Bayón C, Méndez J, Gancedo PG, Grande C, Diez JJ. Serum insulin-like growth factor type 1, insulin-like growth factor-binding protein-1, and insulin-like growth factor-binding protein-3 concentrations in patients with thyroid dysfunction. *Thyroid.* 2001 Nov;11(11):1043-8.

Isogawa K, Haruo Nagayama H, Tsutsumi T, et al. Simultaneous use of thyrotropin-releasing hormone test and combined dexamethasone/corticotropine-releasing hormone test for severity evaluation and outcome prediction in patients with major depressive disorder. *Journal of Psychiatric Research* 2005;39:467-473.

Jackson I. The thyroid axis and depression. *Thyroid* 1998;8(10):951-956.

Jenning AS, Ferguson DC, Utiger RD. Regulation of the conversion of thyroxine to triiodothyronine in the perfused rat liver. *J Clin Invest* 1979;64:1614-1623.

Kantor MJ, Leef KH, Bartoshesky L, et al. Admission thyroid evaluation in very-low-birthweight infants: association with death and severe intraventricular hemorrhage. *Thyroid* 2003;13:965-9.

Kaplan MM. The Role of Thyroid Hormone Deiodination in the Regulation of Hypothalamo-Pituitary Function Progress in Neuroendocrinology. *Neuroendocrinology* 1984;38:254-260.

Kaplein EM, Kaplein JS, Chang EI, et al. Thyroxine transfer and distribution in critical nonthyroidal illness, chronic renal failure, and chronic ethanol abuse. *J Clin Endocrinol Metab* 1987;65:606-616.

Kaptein EM, Robinson WJ, et al. Peripheral serum thyroxine, triiodothyronine, and reverse triiodothyronine in the low thyroxine state of acute nonthyroidal illness. A noncompartmental analysis. *J Clin Invest* 1982;69:526-535.

Kirkegaard C, Faber J. Altered serum levels of thyroxine, triiodothyronines and diiodothyronines in endogenous depression. *Acta Endocrinologica* 1981;96:199-207.

Kirkegaard C, Faber J. Free thyroxine and 3,3',5'-triiodothyroidnine levels in cerebralspinal fluid in patetns with endogenous depression. *Acta Endorcinoligca* 1991;124:166-172.

Kirkegaard C. The thyrotropin response to thyrotropin-releasing hormone in endogenous depression. *Psychoneuroendocrinology* 1981;6:189-212.

Kjellman BF, Ljunggren JG, Beck-Friis J, Wetterberg L. Reverse T3 levels in affective disorders. *Psychiatry Research* 1983;10:1-9.

Koenig RJ, Leonard JL, Senator D, Rappaport N, Regulation of thyroxine 5'-deiodinase activity by 3,5,3'-triiodothyronine in cultured rat anterior pituitary cells. *Endocrinology* 1984;115(1):324-329.

Kozlowska L, Rosolowska-Huszcz. Leptin, Thyrotropin, and Thyroid Hormones in Obese/Overweight Women Before and After Two Levels of Energy Deficit. *Endocrine* 2004;24(2):147-153.

Krenning E, et al. Characteristics of active transport of thyroid hormone into rat hepatocytes. *Biochim Biophys Acta* 1981;676:314–320.

Krenning EP, Docter R, Bernard HF, et al. Decreased transport of thyroxine (T4), 3,3 ,5-triiodothyronine (T3) and 3,3 ,5 - triiodothyronine (rT3) into rat hepatocytes in primary culture due to a decrease of cellular ATP content and various drugs. *FEBS Lett* 1982;140:229-233.

Krenning EP, Docter R, Bernard HF,et al. The essential role of albumin in the active transport of thyroid hormones into primary cultured rat hepatocytes. *FEBS Lett* 1979;1;107(1):227-30.

Krotkiewski M, Holm G, Shono N. Small doses of triiodothyronine can change some risk factors associated with abdominal obesity. *Inter J Obesity* 1997;21:922-929.

Krotkiewski M, Holm G, Shono N. Small doses of triiodothyronine can change some risk factors associated with abdominal obesity. *Inter J Obesity* 1997;21:922-929.

Krotkiewski M. Thyroid hormones and treatment of obesity. *Int J of Obesity* 2000;24(2):S116-S119.

Krulich L, Giachetti A, Marchlewska-Koj A, et al. On the role of central norandrenergic and dopaminergic systems in the regulation of TSH secretion in the rat. *Endocrinology* 1977;100:496-505.

Kucharzewski M, Braziewicz J et al. Concentration of selenium in the whole blood and the thyroid tissue of patients with various thyroid diseases. *Biol Trace Elem Res.* 2002 Jul;88(1):25-30.

Kvetny J. Thyroxine binding and cellular metabolism of thyroxine in mononuclear blood cells from patients with anorexia nervosa. *J Endocrinol.* 1983 Sep;98(3):343-50.

Larsen PR, Silva JE, Kaplan MM. Relationship between circulation and intracellular thyroid haomrones: physiological and clinical implications. *Endcor Rev* 1981;2:87.

Leibel RL, Jirsch J. Diminished energy requirements in reduced-obese patients. *Metabolism* 1984;33(2):164-170.

Lema SC, JT Dickey, IR Schultz and P Swanson. Dietary exposure to 2,2´,4,4´-tetrabromodiphenyl ether (PBDE 47) alters thyroid status and thyroid hormone-regulated gene transcription in the pituitary and brain. *Environmental Health Perspectives* 2008;116:1694–1699.

Lim C-F, Bernard BF, De Jong M, et al. A furan fatty acid and indoxyl sulfate are the putative inhibitors of thyroxine hepatocyte transport in uremia. *J Clin Endocrinol Metab* 1993;76:318-324.

Lim C-F, Docter R, Krenning EP, et al. Transport of thyroxine into cultured hepatocytes: effects of mild nonthyroidal illness and calorie restriction in obese subjects. *Clin Endocrinol* (Oxf) 1994;40:79-85.

Lim C-F, Docter R, Visser TJ, Krenning EP, Bernard B, et al. Inhibition of thyroxine transport into cultured rat hepatocytes by serum of non-uremic critically ill patients: Effects of bilirubin and nonesterified fatty acids. *J Clin Endocrinol Metab* 1993;76:1165-1172.

Lim VS, Passo C, Murata Y, Ferrari E, et al. Reduced triiodothyronine content in liver but not pituitary of the uremic rat model: demonstration of changes compatible with thyroid hormone deficiency in liver only. *Endocrinology* 1984;114:280-286.

Linnoila M, Lamberg BA, Potter WZ, Gold PW, Goodwin FK. High reverse T3 levels in manic and unipolar depressed women. *Psychiatry Research* 1982;6:271-276.

Linnoila M, Lamberg BA, Rosberg G, Karonen SL, Welin MG. Thyroid hormones and TSH, prolactin and LH responses to repeated TRH and LRH injections in depressed patients. *Acta Psychiat Scand* 1979;59:536-544.

Lomax P, Kokka N, George R. Thyroid activity following intracerbral injection of morphine in the rat. *Neuroendocrinolgoy* 1970;6(146):152.

Lomenick JP, El-Sayyid M, Smith WJ. Effect of levo-thyroxine treatment on weight and body mass index in children with acquired hypothyroidism. *The Journal of Pediatrics* 2008;152(1):96-100.

Loucks AB, Heath EM. Induction of low-T3 syndrome in exercising women occurs at the threshold of energy availability. *Am J Physiol Regul Integr Comp Physiol* 1994;266: R817-R823.

Lowe J, et al. Effectiveness and safety of T3 (triiodothyronine) therapy for euthyroid fibromyalgia: a double-blind placebo-controlled response-driven crossover study.: *Clinical Bulletin of Myofascial Therapy*, 2(2/3):31-58, 1997.

Lowe JC ,Reichman AJ, Garrison R, Yellin J.. Triiodothyronine (T3) treatment of euthyroid fibromyalgia: a small-n replication of a double-blind placebo-controlled crossover study. *Clinical Bulletin of Myofascial Therapy*, 2(4):71-88, 1997.

Lowe JC, Reichman AJ, Yellin J. The process of change during T3 treatment for euthyroid fibromyalgia: a double-blind placebo-controlled crossover study.: *Clinical Bulletin of Myofascial Therapy*, 2(2/3):91-124, 1997.

Maffei M, et al. Leptin levels in human and rodent: measurement of plasma leptin and ob NAN in obese and weight-reduced subjects. *Nature Medicine* 1995;1;1155-1161.

Magri F, Fioravanti CM, vignati G, et al. Thyroid function in old and very old healthy subjects. *J Endocrinol Invest* 2002;25(10):60–3.

Maldonado LS, Murata GH, Hershman JM, et al. Do thyroid function tests independently predict survival in the critically ill? *Thyroid* 1992;2:119–23.

Manore MM, Berry TE, Skinner JS, Carroll SS. Energy expenditure at rest and during exercise in nonobese female cyclical dieters and in nondieting control subjects. *Am J Clin Nutr* 1991;54:41-6.

Massart F, Massai G, Placidi G, Saggese G. Child thyroid disruption by environmental chemicals. *Minerva Pediatrica* 2004;58(1):47-53.

McCormack PD. Cold stress, reverse T3 and lymphocyte function. *Alaska Med* 1998;40(3):55-62.

Mebis L, Langouche L, Visser TJ, Van den Berghe G. The type II iodothyronine is up-regulated in skeletal muscle during prolonged critical illness. *J Endocrinol Metab* 2007;92(8):3330-3333.

Meeker JD, Calafat AM, Hauser R. Di(2-ethylhexyl) Phthalate Metabolites May Alter Thyroid Hormone Levels in Men. *Environ Health Perspect* 2007;115:1029–1034.

Meier C, et al. Serum thyroid stimulating hormone in assessment of severity of tissue hypothyroidism in patients with overt primary thyroid failure: cross sectional survey. *BMJ*. 2003 Feb 8;326(7384): 311-2.

Melzer D, et al. Association between serum perfluorooctanoic acid (PFOA) and thyroid disease in the U.S. National Health and Nutrition Examination Survey. *Environ Health Perspect*. 2010 May;118(5):686-92.

Lecomte P, Lecureuil N et al. Age modulates effects of thyroid dysfunction on sex hormone binding globulin (SHBG) levels. *Exp Clin Endocrinol Diabetes*. 1995;103(5):339-42.

Meunier N, et al. Basal metabolic rate and thyroid hormones of late-middle-aged and older human subjects: the ZENITH study. *Eur J Clin Nutr*. 2005 Nov;59 Suppl 2:S53-7.

Mi kiewicz P, K pczy ska-Nyk A, Bednarczuk T. Coeliac disease in endocrine diseases of autoimmune origin. *Endokrynol Pol*. 2012;63(3):240-9.

Mitchell AM, Manley SW, Rowan KA, Mortimer RH. Uptake of reverse T3 in the human choriocarcinoma cell line, JAr. *Placenta*. 1999 Jan;20(1):65-70.

Moriyama K, Tagami T, Akamizu T, Usui T, et al. Thyroid hormone action is disrupted by bisphenol A as an antagonist. *J Clin Endocrin Metab* 2002;87(11):5185-5190.

Morley JE. The endocrinology of the opiates and opioid peptides. *Metabolism* 1981;30(2):195-209.

Nicoloff JT, Fisher DA, Appleman MD. The role of glucocorticoids in the regulation of thyroid function in man. *J Clin Invest*. 1970; 49(10): 1922–1929.

Nierenberg AA, et al. A comparison of lithium and T(3) augmentation following two failed medication treatments for depression: a STAR*D report. *Am J Psychiatry*. 2006 Sep;163(9):1519-30.

Okamoto R, Leibfritz D. Adverse effects of reverse triiodothyronine on cellular metabolism as assessed by 1H and 31P NMR spectroscopy. *Res Exp Med (Berl)*. 1997;197(4):211-7.

Opstad PK, Falch D, Oktedalen O, Fonnum F, Wergeland R. The thyroid function in young men during prolonged exercise and the effect of energy and sleep deprivation. *Clinical Endocrinology* 1984;20:657-669.

Panicker V, Evans J, Bjoro T, Asvold BO. A paradoxical difference in relationship between anxiety, depression and thyroid function in subjects on and not on T4: findings from the Hunt study. *Clinical Endocrinology* 2009;71:574-580.

Panzer C, Wise S, Fantini G, Kang D, et al. Impact of oral contraceptives on sex hormone-binding globulin and androgen levels: a retrospective study in women with sexual dysfunction. *J Sex Med*. 2006 Jan;3(1):104-13.

Papa S. Mitochondrial oxidative phosphorylation changes in the life span. Molecular aspects and physiopathological implications. *Biochimica Biophysica Acta* 1996;87-105.

Peeters RP, Geyten SV, Wouters PJ, et al. Tissue thyroid hormone levels in critical illness. *J Clin Endocrinol Metab* 2005;12:6498–507.

Peeters RP, Wouters PJ, Toor HV, et al. Serum 3,3_,5_-Triiodothyronine (rT3) and 3,5,3_-Triiodothyronine/rT3 Are Prognostic Markers in Critically Ill Patients and Are Associated with Postmortem Tissue Deiodinase Activities. *J Clin Endocrinol Metab* 2005;90(8): 4559–4565.

Premachandra1 BN, Kabir MA, Williams IK. Low T3 syndrome in psychiatric depression. *J Endocrinol Invest* 2006;29: 568-572.

Reed HL, Brice D, Shakir KM, Burman KD, et al. Decreased free fraction of thyroid hormones after prolonged Antarctic residence. *J Applied Physiol* 1990;69:1467-1472.

Richter C. Oxidative damage to mitochondrial DNA and its relationship to aging. *Int J Biochem Cell Biol* 1995;27(7):647-653.

Riley WW, Eales JG. Characterization of 3,5,3-triiodo-lthyronine transport into hepatocytes isolated from juvenile rainbow trout (Oncorhynchus mykiss), and comparison with l-thyroxine transport. *Gen Comp Endocrinol* 1994;95:301–309.

Romaldini JH, Biancalana MM, Figueiredo DI, et al. Effect of L-thyroxine administration on antithyroid antibody levels, lipid profile, and thyroid volume in patients with Hashimoto's thyroiditis. *Thyroid.* 1996; 6: 183-188.

Samuels MH, Schuff KG, Carlson NE, Carello P, Janowsky JS. Health status, psychological symptoms, mood, and cognition in L-thyroxine-treated hypothyroid subjects. *Thyroid* 2007;17(3):249-58.

Santini F, Mantovani A, Cristaudo A, et al. Thyroid function and exposure to styrene. *Thyriod* 2008;18(10):1065-1069.

Sarne DH, Refetoff S, Rosenfield RL, Farriaux JP. Sex hormone-binding globulin in the diagnosis of peripheral tissue resistance to thyroid hormone: the value of changes after short term triiodothyronine administration. *J Clin Endocrinol Metab.* 1988 Apr;66(4):740-6.

Sasano H. Analysis of lectin binding in benign and malignant thyroid nodules. Arch Pathol Lab Med.1989 Feb;113(2):186-9.

Sasano H. An estimation of selenium requirements for New Zealanders. Am J Clin Nutr November 1999 vol. 70 no. 5 896-903.

Schapira AHV. Mitochondrial disease. *Lancet* 2006;368:70-82.

Schilling JU, Zimmermann T, Albrecht S, et al. Low T3 syndrome in multiple trauma patients – a phenomenon or important pathogenetic factor? *Medizinische Klinik* 1999;3:66– 9.

Schulte C, Reinhardt W, Beelen D, et al. Low T3-syndrome and nutritional status as prognostic factors in patients undergoing bone marrow transplantation. *Bone Marrow Transplant* 1998;22:1171– 8.

Selmer C, et al. The spectrum of thyroid disease and risk of new onset atrial fibrillation: a large population cohort study. *BMJ.* 2012 Nov 27;345:e7895.

Sherer TB, Betarbet R, Greenamyre JT. Environment, mitochondria, and Parkinson's disease. *Neuroscientist* 2002;8(3):192–7.

Silva JE, Dick TE, Larsen PR. The contribution of local tissue thyroxine monodeiodination to the nuclear 3,5,3'-triiodothyroinine in pituitary, liver and kidney of euthyroid rats. *Endocrinology* 1978;103:1196. location of D2

Silva JE, Larsen PR 1986 Hormonal regulation of iodothyronine 5-deiodinase in rat brown adipose tissue. *Am J Physiol* 251:E639-E643.

Silva JE, Larsen PR. Pituitary nuclear 3,5,3_-triiodothyronine and thyrotropin secretion: an explanation for the effect of thyroxine. *Science* 1977;198:617–620.

Sintzel F, Mallaret M, Bougerol T. Potentializing of tricyclics and serotoninergics by thyroid hormones in resistant depressive disorders. *Encephale* 2004;30(3):267-75.

Spencer CA, Lum SMC, Wilber JF, et al. Dynamics of Serum Thyrotropin and Thyroid Hormone Changes in Fasting. *J Clin Endocrin Metab* 1983;(5):883-888.

St Germain DL, Galton VA. Comparative study of pituitary-thyroid hormone economy in fasting and hypothyroid rats. *J Clin Invest* 1985,75(2).679-688.

Stavrovskaya IG, Kristal BS. The powerhouse takes control of the cell: is the mitochondrial permeability transition a viable therapeutic target against neuronal dysfunction and death? *Free Radic Biol Med* 2005;38 (6):687–697.

Steen SN, Opplieger RA, Brownell KD. Metabolic effects of repeated weight and regain in adolescent wrestlers. *JAMA* 1988;260:47-50.

Stipcevic T, Pivac N, Kozarie-Kovacic D, Muck-Seler D. Thyroid activity in patients with major depression. *Coll Antropol* 2008;32(3):973-976.

Stump CS, Short KR, Bigelow ML, et al. Effect of insulin on human skeletal muscle mitochondrial ATP production, protein synthesis, and mRNA transcripts. *Proc Natl Acad Sci* 2003;100(13):7996–8001.

Sullivan GM, Hatterer JA, Herbert J, Chen X, Rosse SP. Low levels of transthyretin in CSF of depressed patients. *Am J Psych* 1999;156:710-715.

Szybi ski Z. Iodine prophylaxis in Poland in light of the WHO recommendation on reduction of the daily salt intake. *Pediatr Endocrinol Diabetes Metab.* 2009;15(2):103-7.

Szymanski PT, Effects of thyroid hormones and reverse T3 pretreatment on the betaadrenoreceptors in the rat heart. *Acta Physiol Pol* 1986;37:131-138.

Tennant F. Hormone Treatments in chronic and intractable pain. *Practical Pain Management* 2005; 57-63.

Tetsuyuki Y., et al. Serum vitamin D levels are decreased and associated with thyroid volume in female patients with newly onset Graves' disease. *Endocrine.* 2012 December; 42(3): 739–741.

Thompson FK. Is there a thyroid-cortisol-depression axis? *Thyroid Science* 2007;2(10):1.

Turker O, et al. Selenium treatment in autoimmune thyroiditis: 9-month follow-up with variable doses. *J Endocrinol*. 2006. Jul;190(1):151-6.

Unden F, Ljunggren JG, Kjellman BF, Beck-Friis J, Wetterberg L. Twenty-four-hour serum levels of T4 and T3 in relation to decreased TSH serum levels and decreased TSH response to TRH in affective disorders. *Acta Psychiatr Scand* 1986;73:358-365.

Van der Heyden JT, Docter R, van Toor H, et al. Effects of caloric deprivation on thyroid hormone tissue uptake and generation of low-T3 syndrome. *Am J Physiol Endocrinol Metab* 1986;251(2):156-E163.

van der Poll T, Romijn JA, Wiersinga WM, Sauerwein HP. Tumor necrosis factor: a putative mediator of the sick euthyroid syndrome in man. *J Clin Endo Metab* 1990;71:1567-1572.

Vaughan GM, Mason AD, McManus WF, et al. Alterations of mental status and thyroid hormones after thermal injury. *J Clin Endocrinol Metab* 1985;60:1221–5.

Virili C, Bassotti G, Santaguida MG et al. Atypical celiac disease as cause of increased need for thyroxine: a systematic study. *J Clin Endocrinol Metab*. 2012 Mar;97(3):E419-22.

Visser TJ, Kaplau MM, Leonard JL, Larsen PR. Evidence for two pathways of iodothyroinine 5'-deiodination in rat pituitary that differ I kinetics, propylthiouracil sensitivity, and response to hypothyroidism. *J Clin Invest* 1983;71:992.

Visser TJ, Lamberts WJ, Wilson JHP, Docter WR, Hennemann G. Serum thyroid hormone concentrations during prolonged reduction of dietary intake. *Metabolism* 1978;1978;27(4):405-409.

Visser WE, Friesema EC, Jansen J, Visser TJ. Thyroid hormone transport in and out of cells. *Trends Endocrinol Metab*. 2008 Mar;19(2):50-6.

Vos RA, de Jong M, Bernard BF, et al. Impaired thyroxine and 3,5,3 - triiodothyronine handling by rat hepatocytes in the presence of serum of patients with nonthyroidal illness. *J Clin Endocrinol Metab* 1995;80:2364-2370.

Wassen FWJS, Moerings EPCM, van Toor H, et al. Thyroid hormone uptake in cultured rat anterior pituitary cells: effects of energy status and bilirubin. *J Endocrinol* 2000;165:599-606.

Watanabe C, Yoshida K, Kasanuma Y, Kun Y, Satoh H.. In utero methylmercury exposure differentially affects the activities of selenoenzymes in the fetal mouse brain. *Environ Res* 1999; 80(3):208-14.

Weinsier RL, Nagy TR, Hunter GR, Darnell BE, Hensrud DD, Weiss HL. Do adaptive changes in metabolic rate favor weight regain in weight-reduced individuals? An examination of the set-point theory. *Am J Clin Nutr.* 2000 Nov;72(5):1088-94.

Wekking EM, Appelhof BC, Fliers E, Schene AH, et al. Cognitive functioning and well-being in euthyroid patients on thyroxine replacement therapy for primary hypothyroidism. *European J Endocrinol* 2005;153:747-753.

Whybrow PC, Coppen A, Prange AJ, Noguera R, Bailey JE. Thyroid function and the response to liothyronine in depression. *Arch Gen Psychiatry* 1972;26:242-245.

Yandell SD, Harvey WC, Fernandes NJ, Barr PW, Feldman M. Radioiodine studies, low serum thyrotropin, and the influence of statin drugs. *Thyroid.* 2008 Oct;18(10):1039-42.

Yellin BA, Reichman AJ, Lowe JC ,The process of Change During T3 Treatment for Euthyroid Fibromyalgia. A Double-Blind Placebo-Controlled Crossover Study. *The Metabolic Treatment of Fibromyalgia.* McDowell Publishing 2000.

Zoeller RT, Bansal R, Parris C. Bisphenol-A, an Environmental Contaminant that Acts as a Thyroid Hormone Receptor Antagonist in Vitro, Increases Serum Thyroxine, and Alters RC3/Neurogranin Expression in the Developing Rat Brain. *Endocrinology* 2005;146(2):607-12.

Index

About the Author

Suzy Cohen, America's Pharmacist™ is a licensed pharmacist and Functional Medicine practitioner. She writes a syndicated health column, "Dear Pharmacist," which circulates to millions of readers each week and you can get this sent to your email for free by signing up for her newsletter at *www.SuzyCohen.com*. Suzy hosts a medical minute on "Know the Cause" television and is a Huffington Post blogger. You have seen her on The Dr. Oz Show, The View, The Doctors, Good Morning America Health and hundreds of other television networks. Suzy is also the Founder of ScriptEssentials.com, a company specializing in unique, bio-active nutritional supplements. Suzy is a member of the following organizations:

> *The American College for Advancement in Medicine* (ACAM)
> *The Institute of Functional Medicine* (IFM)
> *The American Academy of Anti-Aging Medicine* (A4M)
> *American Pharmacist's Association* (APhA)
> *International Lyme and Associated Diseases Society* (ILADS)
> *The Academy of Comprehensive Integrative Medicine* (ACIM)

Other Books by Suzy Cohen, RPh:
> *Headache Free: Relieve Migraine, Tension, Cluster, Menstrual and Lyme Headaches* (DPI 2013)
> *The 24-Hour Pharmacist: Advice, Options and Amazing Cures from America's Most Trusted Pharmacist* (Collins 2009)

Diabetes Without Drugs, The 5-Step Program to Control Blood Sugar Naturally and Prevent Diabetes Complications (Rodale 2010)

Drug Muggers: Which Medications are Robbing Your Body of Essential Nutrients and How to Restore Them (Rodale 2011)

Eczema: Itchin' for a Cure (DPI 2012) Kindle only

Understanding Pancreatitis & Pancreatic Cancer (DPI 2012) Kindle only

---

Are you on the computer?

On Facebook *www.Facebook.com/SuzyCohenRPh* click LIKE
Twitter @SuzyCohen
Pinterest: *www.pinterest.com/suzycohen*
